Palliative Nursing

For Baillière Tindall:

Senior Commissioning Editor: Ninette Premdas
Project Development Manager: Dinah Thom
Project Manager: Jane Dingwall
Design Direction: George Ajayi

Palliative Nursing: Bringing Comfort and Hope

Edited by

Shaun Kinghorn MSc BA(Hons) RGN CertEd RNT RCNT
Senior Lecturer, Cancer and Palliative Care, Marie Curie Centre, Newcastle upon Tyne, UK

Richard Gamlin MPhil RN CertEd FETC DipNurs RNT RCNT
Senior Lecturer, St Benedict's Hospice, Monkwearmouth Hospital, Sunderland, UK

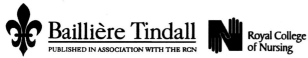

Baillière Tindall
PUBLISHED IN ASSOCIATION WITH THE RCN

Royal College
of Nursing

EDINBURGH LONDON NEW YORK PHILADELPHIA ST LOUIS SYDNEY TORONTO 2001

BAILLIÈRE TINDALL
An imprint of Elsevier Science Limited

 is a registered trademark of Elsevier Science Limited

First published 2001
 Reprinted 2002

0 7020 2422 8

British Library Cataloguing in Publication Data
A catalogue record for this book is available from the British Library

Library of Congress Cataloging in Publication Data
A catalog record for this book is available from the Library of Congress

Note
Medical knowledge is constantly changing. As new information
becomes available, changes in treatment, procedures, equipment and
the use of drugs become necessary. The editors, contributors and
the publishers have taken care to ensure that the information
given in this text is accurate and up to date. However, readers
are strongly advised to confirm that the information, especially
with regard to drug usage, complies with the latest legislation
and standards of practice.

The
publisher's
policy is to use
**paper manufactured
from sustainable forests**

Printed in China by RDC Group Limited

Contents

Contributors

Sally Anstey RNT MSc DipNurs CertEd
ENB237 CertCounselling DipMedEthics
Macmillan Service Development Manager/
Lecturer, University of Wales College of Medicine,
Velindre Hospital NHS Trust, Cardiff, UK

Joanne Atkinson RGN DipHE BA
Senior Lecturer, University of Northumbria at
Newcastle; Palliative Care Team, Leazes Wing,
Royal Victoria Infirmary, Newcastle upon Tyne,
UK

Robert Becker MSc DipN(Lond) RMN RGN
CertEd(FE) FETC730
Macmillan Senior Lecturer, Shropshire and
Mid-Wales Hospice, Bicton Heath, Shrewsbury,
and Staffordshire University School of Health,
Stoke on Trent, UK

Adele Jayne Bird BSc(Hons) RGN RNT PGDE
Director of Education, St Gemma's Hospice,
Leeds, UK

Jacquelyn Chaplin RGN RCNT RNT BA MN
Senior Lecturer, Hunters Hill Marie Curie
Centre, Glasgow, UK

Simon Chippendale MMedSc BSc(Hons) RGN
RNT CertEd DipPallNurs
Senior Lecturer in Palliative Care, St Richard's
Hospice, Worcester, UK

Michael J. Connolly BSc RGN
Macmillan Palliative Care Nurse and Team
Leader, South Manchester University Hospitals
NHS Trust, Manchester, UK

Keith Farrer RGN RNT BA(Hons)
Clinical Nurse Specialist, Palliative Care Team,
Western General Hospital, The Lothian
University Hospitals NHS Trust, Edinburgh, UK

Richard Gamlin MPhil RN CertEd FETC
DipNurs RNT RCNT
Senior Lecturer, St Benedict's Hospice,
Monkwearmouth Hospital, Sunderland, UK

Philippa Green RGN DipHealthStud BSc
CertOncNurs
Clinical Nurse Specialist, Northern Centre for
Cancer Treatment, Newcastle General Hospital,
Newcastle upon Tyne, UK

Shaun Kinghorn MSc BA(Hons) RGN CertEd
RNT RCNT
Senior Lecturer, Cancer and Palliative Care,
Marie Curie Centre, Newcastle upon Tyne, UK

Mel Lewis RGN DippPallNurs BSc
Macmillan Clinical Nurse Specialist, Palliative
Care, Cardiff, UK

Rosemary McIntyre PhD MN RGN
DipN(Lond) NDN(Cert) RNT
Head of Studies (Scotland and Northern
Ireland), Marie Curie Cancer Care (Education),
Edinburgh, UK

Sharon Macnish RN MHHir
Professional Course Director, Selfheal School of
Herbalists, Letchworth Centre for
Complementary Medicine; Director of
Herbalbag, Edinburgh

Angela Mitchell MSc MA BEd(Hons) RNT
RCNT RGN ONC
Senior Lecturer in Palliative Care, University of
Northumbria, Continuing Nurse Education,
Newcastle upon Tyne, UK

Rosie Morton RGN BN(Hons) ENB237,998
CertManagStud PGCE
Head of Education, Butterworth Hospice Care;
Macmillan Lead Nurse for Palliative Care,
County Durham and Darlington Health
Authority, Durham

Sheila Newman MA RMN RGN PG DipEdDev
DipSocRes PGCE
Coordinator/Senior Lecturer, Northern
Palliative Care Network on behalf of Teesside
University, Middlesbrough, UK

Anita Roberts BSc(Hons) DipHE RGN RSCN
Lecturer, Marie Curie Centre, Liverpool,
UK

Christine Searle RGN DipComNurs BSc
Palliative Care Lecturer, Marie Curie Cancer
Care and University of Wales College of
Medicine Cardiff, Penarth, UK

Fiona Setch RGN FETC CTPD CertEd(FE)
ENB934 CertNeuroProg
Staff Development Officer, Marie Curie Centre,
Marie Curie Drive, Newcastle upon Tyne, UK

Alison Virdee MSc AdvDipResMeth RGN
Clinical Nurse Specialist, Palliative Care, Royal
Victoria Infirmary, Newcastle upon Tyne;
Senior Lecturer, Oncology and Palliative Care,
University of Northumbria at Newcastle,
Newcastle upon Tyne, UK

James Youll RGN ONC DipPallCare
ENB100 931 FETC HEFC
Macmillan Nurse, Harton Wing, South
Tyneside General Hospital, Tyne and Wear,
UK

Preface

In 1995 Marie Curie Cancer Care organised a conference in collaboration with St. Oswald's Hospice and the University of Northumbria at Newcastle Upon Tyne, UK. This conference was entitled 'Palliative Care: Bringing Comfort and Hope'. It was this title that heavily influenced not only the title but also the structure of this book. The title deceptively suggests a focus on the art of palliative nursing, but the scientific perspective has been equally represented in this text via the inclusion of evidence-based literature. Some of this evidence can be traced back to contributors' personal research. Case studies, current research, and reflective practice are features of most chapters. Rather than designing another manual of symptom control, the editors acknowledged the existence of excellent texts which are comprehensive in addressing this important topic. We believe the chapters contained in *Palliative Nursing: Bringing Comfort and Hope* help illustrate the contribution of palliative nursing.

This book has been written by nurses for nurses, but is also sensitive to issues which will be of relevance to the practice of disciplines other than nursing. The aim of this text is to offer a foundation for practitioners providing palliative care as all or part of their work. Whilst cancer is the main focus, the editors and contributors believe a significant proportion of this book is relevant to the care of patients with non-malignant disease.

Nurses currently engaged in study at diploma and degree level within the specialty will find that the book complements other books in this area and will help in meeting the requirements of these programmes and giving an orientation to the specialty. This book is divided into three main sections: promoting comfort to patients and their families; supporting patients and their families through meaningful communication; current issues/challenges in palliative nursing.

Section one focuses on pain and symptom control, orthodox and complementary therapies, and spirituality. These issues are examined in relation to the concept of promoting comfort. Section two moves into the domain of psychosocial issues that impact on the role of the nurse from diagnosis to death and beyond. As palliative nursing continues to develop, many contextual and political factors impact on the boundaries of palliative nursing. Section three explores such topical themes as ethics, research, quality of life, and the needs of the disadvantaged dying. The final chapter, 'Looking after Yourself', appropriately deviates from the overall style of text to help readers consider how they can look after themselves. How can we bring comfort and hope to patients and their families if we are not empowered with the skills and self-awareness to promote our own wellbeing?

2000   Shaun Kinghorn and Richard Gamlin

Acknowledgements

We are grateful to the contributors who have not only helped craft this final version but also helped maintain a sense of purpose and much needed enthusiasm for this project. Thank you also to Jane Dingwall, Dinah Thom, Alex Mathieson, and Sarah James, who patiently guided us through the development of this text. We sincerely hope that reading *Palliative Nursing: Bringing Comfort and Hope* will help you wherever you practise.

Shaun Kinghorn and Richard Gamlin

Thank you to my wife, Melanie, who has been my friend and source of inspiration from the very beginning. Thanks also to our children Aaron, Melanie, Ashley, Anna and Joseph who continue to bring joy, comfort, and hope.

I dedicate my contribution to the development of this book to my late brother-in-law, Stuart, who now 'runs and is no longer weary in his fields of gold', also his wife, Katy, and children, Layla, Stu, and Juliette. A special thanks to the Haematology Unit at the RVI, Newcastle upon Tyne, who through skillful and sensitive care of Stuart and his family enlarged my understanding of palliative care.

Thanks also to my education and clinical colleagues within Marie Curie Cancer Care, in particular those whom I work with on a day-to-day basis at the Marie Curie Centre, Newcastle.

Shaun Kinghorn

Bringing comfort to patients and their families

SECTION CONTENTS

1

Palliative nursing: past, present and future

Richard Gamlin

It is easy to forget how short is the history of Palliative Care and how much has been achieved in that time. It is rapidly becoming an established feature of health care provision in the United Kingdom, understood and employed by some but misunderstood, suspected and resented by others. It has developed and continues to develop in a climate of immensely rapid change. This change is part clinical, part social, both national and international and part related to the organisation of health care. It is influenced by changing expectations and responses, fluctuating economic and political priorities and increasing materialism and technical developments all taking place in a society uncomfortable with loss in any form yet surrounded by it on all sides.   (Doyle 1997)

This chapter outlines the history and development of palliative care, comments on present-day issues and looks to the future. As palliative care aims to provide holistic care for patients and those who matter to them it would be arrogant to refer solely to nursing and nurses without acknowledging multi-professional teamwork and the enormous contribution made by volunteers. Saunders said, in 1959, 'The care of the dying is pre-eminently the time for the doctor, nurse and chaplain to co-operate, at a time when they have a responsibility to do the best they can for the people who turn to them' (Saunders 1960). Today we would add many more members of the multi-professional team to the short list above as physiotherapists, occupational therapists, dieticians, pharmacists and complementary therapists establish their rightful place in the palliative care team.

This chapter does not discuss in detail the history of palliative care, as this has been done so well by others although a brief history is included so that the reader can judge the impact of history on today's practice. Many of the issues raised in this chapter are discussed in depth in the following chapters. Some topics not covered as discrete chapters are introduced in this chapter, notably international palliative care and the often neglected issue of sexuality.

A BRIEF HISTORY OF PALLIATIVE CARE

Originally hospices were not concerned with dying. The word 'hospice' comes from the Latin *hospes* meaning a host. Hospices became places of pilgrimage based on Christian principles. From the medieval hospices where travellers found rest came the modern Catholic hospice. In 1879 Our Lady's Hospice in Dublin was founded, followed in 1900 by St Joseph's Hospice in East London. In 1948 the Marie Curie Memorial Foundation began caring for patients with advanced cancer. They began their work by opening terminal care homes throughout the United Kingdom.

Macmillan Cancer Relief, formerly Cancer Relief Macmillan Fund, was formed after Douglas Macmillan, aged 27, watched his father die of cancer. He was shocked and surprised to find how little doctors appeared to know about caring for patients with cancer. He discovered that the public knew even less about cancer. The charity began as the Society for the Prevention and Relief of Cancer. Its aim was to inform professionals and the public about cancer. The charity was not welcomed by all. In the early 1920s the charity expanded its work to help families cope with cancer. In 1924 the charity distributed £11 in grants to patients while in 1998, Macmillan Cancer Relief gave £5.1 million in grants.

Macmillan Cancer Relief now funds Macmillan nurses, doctors and other health care professionals in careful partnership with the National Health Service. It continues to make financial grants to patients and families and makes larger grants to fund the development of palliative care buildings and services.

In 1959, while Cicely Saunders was a research fellow at St. Mary's Hospital she wrote a series of articles about the care of the dying. These were later published by *Nursing Times* (Saunders 1960) and received favourable reviews by the *Lancet* and the *Manchester Guardian* (Clark 1997). In 1967 St. Christopher's Hospice was founded in Sydenham, London in recognition of the fact that the needs of the dying were not being met, and the principles of palliative care were established. These principles were that palliative care should be:

* holistic
* multidisciplinary
* scientifically based
* meeting the needs of the patient and family
* emphasising high professional standards
* research based
* evaluative
* providing education and training.

Florence Wald spent a sabbatical year at St. Christopher's, during 1968, and went on to develop hospice care in America's first hospice, the Connecticut Hospice. Elisabeth Kubler-Ross published her influential book *On Death and Dying* in 1969. In this book she said, 'We live in a very particular death denying society. We isolate both the dying and the old and it serves a purpose. They are reminders of our own mortality'. She campaigned for better home care together with emotional, spiritual and financial support. Although many have criticised Kubler-Ross for what they regard as her inflexible approach to loss and grief, few can deny the major contribution she has made to opening up the death-denying society by encouraging lay persons and professionals to talk about death and loss. Indeed, today, it is difficult to find a student of health care who is unable to quote, *or misquote* her work.

The Standing Medical Advisory Committee, in 1980, under the chairmanship of Professor Eric Wilkes warned against the unplanned development of palliative care services in favour of education and support. He urged caution for those well-meaning groups of people keen to have a hospice on every street corner. To some extent his warning was heard and heeded but many services began as a result of public enthusiasm, some with a religious foundation, but few were planned on the basis of local need or with thought to subsequent budgeting and staffing implications. The rapid increase in the provision of palliative care beds appears to have slowed down but in the year 2001 we are still seeing a rise in children's palliative care services. I may not be forgiven for criticising such developments but my concerns reflect those of Professor Wilkes. Those developing services must establish a need before embarking on costly building and subsequently staffing and running costs.

PALLIATIVE CARE: RECENT HISTORY AND THE PRESENT DAY

The last decade has brought palliative care through rapid change and growth. In 1985 there were less than 100 hospices in the UK and now there are over 200 with over 400 home care teams compared with less than 50 in 1985.

In the early 1980s palliative nursing became a specialty. The English National Board for Nursing, Midwifery and Health Visiting approved the development of palliative nursing courses, notably the ENB 931 and 285. At first these courses attracted nurses working in hospices, specialist palliative care services and oncology units. Later they were to attract nurses working in non-specialist units although, even today, the nurse working in an intensive therapy unit may find it hard to persuade his/her manager of the relevance of a palliative care course to a critical care unit. Today an impressive and bewildering array of palliative care education is available from short courses to conferences through to diploma, first and higher degrees. Palliative care is the focus of some doctoral research studies.

The Diploma in Palliative Medicine from the University of Wales which began over 10 years ago has attracted doctors from hospices, hospitals and general practice. Many of those attending this course are from the United Kingdom but it also attracts doctors from Europe, Scandinavia and the Far East. The demand for

this course remains high and some of its graduates go on to become palliative care consultants while others enhance and influence palliative care as non-specialists.

As well as the above unidisciplinary courses, multidisciplinary palliative care courses are emerging: for example, the Masters in Palliative Care at Southampton University. Challenges remain in attempting to enhance multidisciplinary working through education but palliative care attempts to lead the way by example. My local health authority has taken a fresh approach to multidisciplinary palliative care education. All staff from one or two general practices including non-clinical staff come together on two separate occasions to learn about palliative care. The first session focuses on communication issues and teamwork and the second on clinical challenges. No attempt is made to address every problem that they may ever face as a team. On the contrary, the team are encouraged to identify challenges *and* ways of meeting those challenges. The administrative and clerical staff have been instrumental in finding solutions to common problems.

The Association of Palliative Medicine for Great Britain was born in 1985 in recognition of the fact that palliative care was a medical specialty in its own right. Two years later *Palliative Medicine*, the first peer-reviewed professional journal in the field, was launched and the European Association for Palliative Care was formed. In the same year palliative medicine was recognised as a medical specialty with its own training programme. As the specialty developed, more patients were referred earlier and, employing the principles of rehabilitation, more patients were discharged from hospices and palliative care units. In the United Kingdom, in the year 2000, there was a worrying shortage of senior palliative care doctors who have completed specialist training and are ready to take up consultant posts despite the attractive nature and favourable working conditions offered. The Association of Palliative Medicine has worked and is working very hard to remedy this situation although palliative care services will have to weather this storm for the foreseeable future.

Hospices' palliative care units and palliative care teams developed in exactly the way Professor Wilkes had warned against. One worrying consequence of this, coupled with the internal market developing in the National Health Service (NHS), was that hospices were competing with each other for their funds and therefore their very existence. During the late 1990s some senior staff from the independent hospices became concerned that their voice was not being heard at national level. Against the better judgement of some senior clinicians and managers the Independent Hospices Representatives Committee (IHRC) was formed. This body aims to represent the independent hospices but there is much scope for duplication of effort and bureaucracy. Each NHS region now has a National Council for Hospice and Specialist Palliative Care Services (NCHSPCS) representative and an IHRC representative. Those who raise funds for the independent hospices and the large cancer charities could be forgiven for asking if the money they raise is being spent wisely. Indeed they have a right to know, as the trustees have a responsibility to spend wisely.

In 1991 the National Council for Hospice and Specialist Palliative Care Services and the Scottish Partnership Agency for Palliative and Cancer Care were formed, bringing together under one umbrella organisation representatives from all the many professional organisations formed in the previous few years; the NHS and voluntary sectors, the national charities, and, through elected regional representatives, all palliative care providers. Organisations and bodies represented on the National Council for Hospice and Specialist Palliative Care Services and Scottish Partnership Agency include:

- Association of Hospice Chaplains
- Association of Hospice Volunteer Co-ordinators
- Association of Nurse Teachers in Palliative Care
- Macmillan Cancer Relief
- Marie Curie Cancer Care
- Association of Hospice and Specialist Palliative Care Social Workers
- Royal College of Nursing Palliative Nursing Forum
- Association of Palliative Medicine
- Association of Hospice Administration
- Help the Hospices
- Sue Ryder Foundation
- Forum of Chairmen of Independent Hospices
- Scottish Motor Neurone Disease Association
- The Leukaemia Care Association
- The Malcolm Sargent Cancer Fund for Children.

The *Oxford Textbook of Palliative Medicine*, edited by Doyle et al, was first published in 1993. This established the first major authoritative textbook with contributions from all health care disciplines and from many countries around the world. The *European Journal of Palliative Care* was first published in 1994 followed by the *International Journal of Palliative Nursing* in 1995, while 1996 saw the establishment of the first chairs of palliative medicine and palliative care in the United Kingdom.

Table 1.1 Hospices and palliative care services in the UK and Ireland

	Total units	Total beds	NHS units	NHS beds	Voluntary units	Voluntary beds
England	158	2514	36	446	122	2068
Wales	13	124	10	68	3	56
Scotland	24	345	10	86	14	259
N Ireland	4	65			4	65
Ireland	10	136			10	136
Channel Islands and Isle of Man	3	21				21
Total	212	3205	56	600	156	2605

In January 2000 the Hospice Information Service at St. Christopher's identified the hospices and palliative care services in the United Kingdom and the Republic of Ireland (Table 1.1). The number of beds per unit ranges from 2 to 63 (average 15). The total of services includes 19 children's hospices with 145 beds in total and three services for patients with HIV/AIDS (74 beds). In addition to hospice units there are other services (Table 1.2).

The two largest cancer charities in the United Kingdom make an enormous contribution to palliative care. Marie Curie Cancer Care has 10 inpatient centres and over 6000 Marie Curie nurses who care for people in their own homes during the day or night. Marie Curie Cancer Care also has a research institute concentrating on molecular aspects of cancer. It collaborates with many international cancer research organisations. Marie Curie Cancer Care has a large educational team providing cancer and palliative care education to all health care professionals and volunteers.

Macmillan Cancer Relief aims to help improve the quality of life for patients with cancer. It funds Macmillan nurses and doctors, builds cancer care units and gives grants to patients and their families. Medical support and education for the Macmillan nurses and doctors is a key feature of the organisation. Macmillan general practice facilitators are general practitioners who spend part of their working week enhancing cancer care in the local community.

Both organisations work closely with the NHS and to some extent work together. If both are to continue to grow and develop they will need to examine their working relationships and their strategic direction if they are to make best use of charitable donations and avoid duplication of effort.

In 1990 the World Health Organization defined palliative care as follows:

the active total care of patients whose disease no longer responds to curative treatment. Control of pain, of other symptoms and of psychological, social and spiritual problems is paramount. The goal of palliative care is achievement of the best quality of life for patients and their families.

Their definition continued by stating that palliative care:

- affirms life and regards dying as a normal process
- neither hastens or postpones death
- provides relief from pain and other distressing symptoms
- integrates the psychological and spiritual aspects of patient care
- offers a support system to help patients live as actively as possible until death
- offers a support system to help the family to cope during the patient's illness and into their own bereavement.

The National Council for Hospice and Specialist Palliative Care Services (1997) presented the following principles which underpin palliative care provision:

It is the right of every person with a life-threatening illness to receive palliative care wherever they are.
It is the responsibility of every health care professional to practice the palliative care approach, and to call in specialist palliative care colleagues if

Table 1.2 Services other than hospice units in the UK and Ireland

	Home care	Extended home care	Day care	Hospital support teams	Hospital support nursing services
England	258	48	195	165	96
Wales	29	5	16	23	2
Scotland	42	7	19	21	14
N Ireland	9	1	4	6	6
Ireland	26	3	6	11	4
Channel Islands and Isle of Man	3	2	3	0	1
Total	367	66	243	226	123

the need arises, as an integral component of good clinical practice, whatever the illness or its stage.

If these rights and responsibilities are to be achieved and sustained, health care professionals must be empowered and enabled to fulfil their responsibilities. The principles of palliative care for all will need to be integrated into the whole of the NHS, to include patients with non-malignant disease and patients with learning disabilities and mental health problems. This will take commitment from health authorities, primary care groups and trusts who commission care down to the individual practitioner who delivers care. It can be achieved but will be an evolutionary rather than a revolutionary process.

The NCHSPCS (1999) defined the palliative care approach:

The palliative care approach aims to promote both physical and psychosocial well-being. It is a vital and integral part of all clinical practice, whatever the illness or its stage, informed by a knowledge and practice of palliative care principles and supported by specialist palliative care. The key principles underpinning palliative care which should be practised by all health care professionals in primary care, hospital and other settings comprise:

- focus on quality of life which includes good symptom control
- whole person approach taking into account the person's life experience and current situation
- care which encompasses both the patient and those who matter to that person
- respect for patient autonomy and choice (e.g. over place of care, treatment options, access to specialist palliative care)
- emphasis on open and sensitive communication which extends to patients, informal carers and professional colleagues.

The definition of the palliative care approach has been enormously helpful in clarifying the individual and collective responsibilities of health care professionals. Many who encounter the definition for the first time are readily convinced of its universal applicability. The palliative care approach forms the basis of much ward/team care philosophy and serves as an excellent basis for foundation courses in palliative care. Health care professionals regard the palliative care approach as their responsibility

and strive to integrate it into their practice. In so doing inappropriate referrals to specialist palliative care teams are likely to decrease.

Specialist palliative care will be required by a proportion of patients with cancer and life-threatening illnesses who are unable to be managed using the palliative care approach. According to the NCHSPCS (1999):

Specialist palliative care is the active total care of patients with progressive far advanced illness and limited prognosis, and their families, by a multi-professional team who have undergone recognised specialist palliative care training. It provides physical, psychological, social and spiritual support, and will involve practitioners with a broad mix of skills, including medical and nursing, social work, pastoral/spiritual care, physiotherapy, occupational therapy, pharmacy and related specialities.

Stjernsward (1993) said:

Nothing would have greater impact than to act on the knowledge we already have. Nothing would have greater impact on the future of palliative care than the universal acceptance of and commitment to the palliative care approach.

PALLIATIVE CARE: INTERNATIONAL ISSUES

No chapter addressing the past, present and future of palliative care would be complete without considering palliative care in developing countries. It was Stjernsward, in 1993, who said: 'No effective palliative care is available to the eight or nine out of ten patients in developing countries that are already incurable at the time of diagnosis'. It is not the author's intention to describe palliative care in all developing countries but to illustrate some of the problems faced by those who are attempting to provide palliative care to large numbers of the world's population. For further information, see Saunders & Kastenbaum (1997) and Clark et al (1997).

The challenges that face those providing palliative care in developing countries go beyond opioid availability and restricted access to suitable cancer treatment facilities. Open, sensitive communication, one of the key elements of the palliative care approach, is difficult in cultures where everyday communication is, or has been historically, charged with problems. The UK reader should remember that open, sensitive communication was not commonly practised in the UK health care system until the last decade of the second millennium and indeed today there is much room for improvement.

Russia provides an example of the types of problems faced by patients, families and health care professionals in developing countries. It is important to remember that each country may have its own unique problems. Jones (1997) describes the cultural issues in Russia that influence the delivery of palliative care. Russia's past and recent history is that of ordinary people who have reserved their innermost thoughts and feelings for their immediate family and a small circle of intimate friends. It is hard for Russians today to trust each other, their politicians and indeed their health professionals. Many British-run courses have been delivered throughout the former Soviet Union with the aim of encouraging Russian health professionals to adopt the palliative care approach. Open and sensitive communication is perhaps the most difficult principle for them to subscribe to.

Becker (1999), while teaching at the First Moscow Hospice in 1997, found himself in a situation which required the utmost skill and judgement. He describes the care of Alexander, an elderly Russian gentleman with advanced cancer. Their discussion through a skilled interpreter led Becker to believe that Alexander wanted to know the truth. Becker had to decide whether to go along with the collusion that had been developing throughout Alexander's illness or to answer Alexander's request for information with honesty and sensitivity. Becker listened to his head and his heart and confirmed what Alexander already knew. This demonstrates how it is possible to overcome many of the challenges identified by Jones (1997) with an honest sensitive approach to communicating with the dying.

British Aid For Hospices Abroad (BAHA) is a small British organisation whose members meet to discuss overseas projects designed to assist in the establishment of palliative care in developing countries. Most of BAHA's members have funded their own projects and have made a significant impact on palliative care in the developing world.

SEXUALITY AND PALLIATIVE CARE

When planning this book the editors and contributors met to discuss the content. Their aim was to present an holistic text without attempting to break down holism into its constituent parts, thus fragmenting an essentially integrated concept. Much discussion arose about whether or not to include a discrete chapter on sexuality. It was decided that, where applicable, each chapter would address the concept. If we claim to provide holistic care we simply cannot ignore sexuality.

In the first chapter of the book the author wishes to alert the reader to the importance of sexuality in those facing advanced illness. Roper et al (1980) were responsible for alerting UK nurses to sexuality when they presented their activities of living model of nursing. One of the activities is expressing sexuality. In 1987, Savage discussed nurses, gender and sexuality in a way that established addressing sexuality as a nursing responsibility. Savage interviewed a student nurse who said:

> We use Roper's model. We go through all of them, in class, and *in theory* it's very good. One of those is expressing sexuality and that's important. But when it comes to doing it in class, what do you talk about? Helping women to look better after they've had their hysterectomy so their husbands will want to have sex with them? You spend ages on breathing then you get to the end of the list, dying and expressing sexuality, and how we should talk to patients and get them to express their feelings, and that's it. No-one ever does it! We write in our care plans 'Encourage questions and help patients to express their feelings and anxieties', but it's never really approached.

When teaching about sexuality the author presents the above quotation to the group without the date of the quotation and invites them to guess when this was written. Most students agree that it could have been written yesterday rather than in 1987, implying that little has changed. Sutherland & Gamlin (1999) discussed body image and sexuality and their implications for those receiving and providing palliative care. They offer many practical suggestions for addressing sexuality in palliative care. Most patients do not require the assistance of a psychosexual counsellor but simply need someone to listen to their concerns and to offer simple advice. The P-LI-SS-I-T model (Annon 1976) is described by Sutherland & Gamlin (1999) and Gamlin (1999). This model, although originally designed to facilitate re-adjustment following myocardial infarction, has been used in palliative care.

The P-LI-SS-I-T model of sexual readjustment

Permission

The nurse gives permission to the patient to talk about worries or concerns. This may involve asking direct questions or being available and accessible.

Limited Information

Factual general information is given about the condition and how this may affect the patient's feeling and functioning. For example what to expect after pelvic surgery *and* how to cope with it.

Specific Suggestions

More in-depth information may be required. A knowledge of relevant anatomy, physiology and pathology will help. Specific information relating to specific cancers will be given.

Intensive Therapy

Some patients and their partners may require intensive therapy, i.e. referral to a psychosexual counsellor but, if the preceding steps are followed, it is likely that most patients' needs can be met without specialist referral.

Health care in the United Kingdom is not yet ready for double beds in institutions, although occasionally this has been arranged. Sexual relationships are and will remain deeply private but, if we are to deliver truly holistic palliative care, we must provide an environment where patients and their partners feel able to express their concerns in the knowledge that they will be met with skill, tact, diplomacy and confidentiality. For the patients who are soon to die and their partners who are soon to be bereaved we must help them to make the best of the life that is left and enhance opportunities for cherished memories.

Even today cancer and death are still often muttered in hushed tones, and fear and ignorance abound. The media are generally sensitive and supportive to hospice and palliative care but may still misrepresent reality.

A recent article entitled 'Welcome to your NHS Death Machine', in a popular magazine said: 'Every day people are given this device on the National Health. It is a syringe driver, a computerised box linked to a tube. You can kill yourself with it. If you are too weak then a friend or relative can press the button for you'. The two-page spread carried photographs of Dr Jack Kevorkian currently serving a jail sentence for second-degree murder in the United States and Dr David Moor charged with murdering a patient with advanced cancer and heart disease, but not convicted. The implication of this article was that euthanasia is regularly carried out in the UK and abroad but the authorities do not own up to it.

Articles like this, although 5-minute wonders, can cause immense distress to patients who are dying and to the bereaved. They misrepresent the reality of palliative care, which continues to strive for the best quality of life for those who are dying and bereaved. Those who are passionate about palliative care have much to be pleased about and indeed proud of but, if we are to strive for palliative care for all, there is no time to rest on our laurels.

THE FUTURE OF PALLIATIVE CARE

Having looked at some of the issues that have affected the development of palliative care and its present state, the chapter now draws to a close by pondering the future of palliative care. The future is presented as a series of predictions that are intended to provoke thought and reflection:

- Specialist palliative care services will continue to grow, albeit more slowly than before. The growth will take into consideration demographic changes and disease development. Specialists will take on a facilitative supportive role rather than be primary providers of care.
- Because of ever-increasing competition, palliative care services will find it difficult to raise sufficient funds to support their development and sustain their provision.
- Children's palliative care services will continue to grow but must be based on need rather than emotion.
- Palliative care will become increasingly available to patients with non-malignant disease. This will not be achieved by building more hospices for end-stage cardiac disease or extending existing buildings to accommodate ever-increasing patient numbers. This will be achieved through effective needs analysis, cooperation, consultation and education.
- Palliative care will grow in the developing countries. This will largely be achieved by the efforts of a small group of committed individuals. A little money will go a long way and the developed countries will accept their responsibility to help those less fortunate than themselves.
- All health care professionals will come to accept the principles of palliative care as part of their daily work.
- Palliative care will become a taught and examined component of all undergraduate health care programmes.
- Specialist palliative care, despite ethical and practical challenges, will become evidence-based.

- Cooperation *must* replace competition in all aspects of palliative care delivery, research and education.

This chapter began with a quotation from Derek Doyle. It will end with some reflections on the memories and musings of this great teacher. Doyle's (1999) book, *The Platform Ticket*, should be read by every health care professional and student of health care. If they read nothing else they would understand the true meaning of palliative care.

When teaching palliative care to a non-specialist audience one sometimes meets a verbal or non-verbal stone wall. Enquiries receive responses such as 'It's alright for you in this well-staffed hospice with all modern facilities but where we work ...'. Working in a hospice undoubtedly brings its perks and privileges but 'having time' brings with it opportunities to discover more patients' problems in more detail and this is how it should be. Doyle (1999) reminds us that experience shows, beyond any possible doubt, that people coming to the end of their lives want quality time rather than a long time. Just a few minutes can be enough if the carer is prepared to sit, listen and answer questions honestly and without jargon.

My final reflection, having taught palliative care for many years, leads me to conclude that I have so much more to learn. Despite an enormous provision of palliative care education, much remains to be done. Most students come along desperately wanting to improve the care of the dying patients they serve: some come with unrealistic expectations. If a teacher advertises a series of study days or sessions about palliative care the pain and symptom study days are always more popular than the loss, grief and communication. This is for two reasons. First, it is easier to teach facts and we may find it easier to focus on the more tangible aspects of care. Evidence-based care, although an important part of palliative care, does not hold all the answers. Secondly, students come looking for the holy grail of palliative care, expecting to find it in the shape of a new drug or drug delivery method. Although new drugs are slowly appearing, those which we already have and understand well are quite capable of controlling most pain, *in the hands of skilled practitioners.*

In the words of Pushkin: 'Education does not mean teaching people to know what they do not know; it means teaching them to behave as they do not behave'. As well as satisfying the thirst for knowledge we must continue to strive for ways of enhancing palliative care through more effective education. This is the future of palliative care.

REFERENCES

Annon J 1976 The behavioural treatment of sexual problems: brief therapy. Harper and Rowe, New York

Becker R 1999 Adult/elderly care nursing. Teaching communication with the dying across cultural boundaries. British Journal of Nursing 8(14): 938–942

Clark D 1997 Someone to watch over me. Nursing Times 93(34): 50–52

Clark D, Hockley J, Ahmedzai S (eds) 1997 New themes in palliative care. Open University Press, Buckingham

Doyle D 1997 Dilemmas and direction: the future of specialist palliative care. A discussion paper. National Council for Hospice and Specialist Palliative Care Services

Doyle D 1999 The platform ticket. Memories and musings of a hospice doctor. Pentland, Durham

Doyle D, Hanks G W, Macdonald N (eds) 1993 The Oxford textbook of palliative medicine. Oxford University Press, Oxford

Gamlin R D 1999 Sexuality: a challenge for nursing practice. Nursing Times 95(7): 48–51

Hospice Information Service 2000 Directory. Hospice and Palliative Care Services in the UK and Republic of Ireland. St. Christopher's Hospice, London

Jones W 1997 Issues affecting the delivery of palliative care in Russia. International Journal of Palliative Nursing 3(2): 82–86

NCHSPCS 1997 Occasional paper 11. Dilemmas and directions. The future of specialist palliative care. National Council for Hospice and Specialist Palliative Care Services, London

NCHSPCS 1999 Palliative care 2000. Commissioning through partnership. National Council for Hospice and Specialist Palliative Care Services, London

Roper N, Logan W, Tierney A 1980 The elements of nursing. Churchill Livingstone, Edinburgh

Saunders C 1960 Care of the dying. Nursing Times, London

Saunders C, Kastenbaum R (eds) 1997 Hospice care on the international scene. Springer, New York

Savage J (ed.) 1987 Nurses gender and sexuality. Heinemann, London

Standing Medical Advisory Committee 1980 Terminal care: report of a working group (the Wilkes report). HMSO, London

Stjernsward J 1993 Palliative medicine – a global perspective. In: Doyle D, Hanks G W, Macdonald N (eds) Oxford textbook of palliative medicine. Oxford University Press, Oxford

Sutherland N, Gamlin R D 1999 Body image and sexuality: implications for palliative care. In: Lugton J, Kindlen M (eds) Palliative care: the nursing role. Churchill Livingstone, Edinburgh

WHO 1990 Cancer pain relief and palliative care. Technical report series 804. World Health Organization, Geneva

2

Pain control

Keith Farrer

INTRODUCTION

Pain is synonymous with cancer in the eyes of the public, and in many cases, in the mind-set of the health care professional.

Yet the World Health Organization (WHO 1996) reports that it is possible to achieve good pain control in the majority of patients with cancer pain. Studies that have systematically applied the World Health Organization's (WHO 1996) guidelines for cancer pain management have achieved adequate pain management in up to 90% of patients (Ventafridda et al 1987, Grond et al 1996). However, outside of such studies, reports of cancer pain management in clinical areas highlight that this level of pain management is not achieved. Recent studies (Bonica 1990, Cleeland 1994), still reveal that approximately one-third to one-half of cancer patients needlessly experience moderate to severe pain (McCaffery & Ferrell 1997).

Disappointingly, these figures are present despite the concerted efforts of both educationalists (in nursing and medicine) and the specialist palliative care movements' push to improve the standards of pain management in clinical areas.

WHY IS CANCER PAIN UNDER-MANAGED?

It is likely that the reasons for this apparent difficulty in achieving adequate pain control for cancer patients are multifaceted and multidisciplinary. Recent literature in nursing and medicine points to a multitude of factors which impinge on our ability to deal with cancer pain adequately (Twycross 1994, McCaffery & Ferrell 1997, Paice et al 1998). These include:

- poor knowledge of cancer pain management
- inappropriate attitudes (i.e. cancer pain is inevitable)
- Poor clinical skills (particularly in the assessment of pain)
- Inappropriate beliefs regarding the management of cancer pain (fears of addiction and tolerance to opiates)
- A lack of appreciation of the non-physical manifestations of cancer pain.

Although the above attitudes, beliefs and skills impact on the management of cancer pain, there are undoubtedly difficulties associated with individual patients that compound the problem. These may include patients with:

- low expectations of pain management and a belief that pain is inevitable
- inappropriate beliefs regarding pain management strategies (i.e. fear of addiction and tolerance)
- beliefs that side effects of medications are inevitable (i.e. sedation).

These difficulties may lead to patients under-reporting pain and result in difficulties with drug compliance.

This chapter attempts to deal with many of these issues, focusing mainly on achievable strategies of cancer pain management. The alleviation of distress is synonymous with achieving hope for a better quality of life, particularly for those patients in whom the focus of treatment is not curative. Achieving this aim is paramount for nursing and should be the focus of nursing interventions in all clinical settings – hospital, hospice or community. Throughout the following paragraphs the main focus is on nursing practice that endeavours to achieve comfort for patients with pain, but it is also recognised that in clinical practice this endeavour needs to be multidisciplinary.

Although nurses have a pivotal role to play in achieving this outcome, it cannot be done with-out good interdisciplinary teamwork. Moreover, it must not be assumed that the attitudes and skills outlined in this chapter are the sole preserve of the nursing profession. In practice there is much overlap of roles and a need for all health care disciplines to attain the core skills for cancer pain management.

It is not the intention to provide an authoritative text in all areas relating to cancer pain management in nursing. Rather, the emphasis will be on strategies that are most likely to produce positive outcomes and, at the same time, be achievable within clinical settings.

In recognition that different clinical contexts require differing levels of skills within nursing, I have split the chapter into the following two areas:

- Part 1. Standard practice—what every nurse needs to know
- Part 2. Higher level of practice.

This structure is based on the premise that all nurses should achieve a core level of knowledge and skill in pain management for patients requiring palliative care. However, in specific clinical areas (such as in oncology and specialist palliative care settings) where a major component of nursing is pain management, there is a requirement for a higher level of practice (UKCC 1999).

PART 1: STANDARD PRACTICE – WHAT EVERY NURSE NEEDS TO KNOW

UNDERSTANDING PAIN

An initial function of pain is to protect and warn that something is not as it should be. Pain undoubtedly protects us from serious injury (such as touching something that is hot), and in the context of illness is often a presenting feature that leads a person to seek medical advice. However, beyond this function, pain becomes less useful and, in chronic illness, becomes debilitating and a source of constant distress. The focus of this chapter is on pain that has long since ceased to serve as a protective mechanism for a person with an illness that is life threatening (such as cancer) and not amenable to curative treatment.

There have been several attempts, none of which is completely satisfactory, to explain and define pain. Perhaps the most recognised definition of pain, is that it is:

an unpleasant sensory and emotional experience associated with actual or potential tissue damage, or described in terms of such damage.   (IASP 1986)

This definition, arrived at by a multidisciplinary expert committee, begins to hint at the possibility of pain being more than just a physical experience, but does not go far enough in encapsulating the total experience or the consequences of unrelieved pain. Pain, associated with an underlying life-threatening and chronic illness, has emotional and spiritual components and often limits the social functioning of the patient, family and friends.

It is not uncommon to hear both the health care professional and the lay person discussing a person's pain in terms of a low- or high-pain threshold. In a clinical situation this is not a useful discussion, as it is unhelpful in the management of the person's pain. Moreover, a patient's supposedly low-pain threshold may be used to excuse poor pain management.

Contrary to popular beliefs, pain thresholds, defined as 'the least experience of pain a person can recognise' (IASP 1986), are remarkably similar amongst healthy volunteers and across different cultures (Bowsher 1993, Twycross 1994). A more important concept is that of pain tolerance (the greatest level of pain which a person is prepared to put up with in a given circumstance or context – see Box 2.1 for definitions related to this area). Bowsher (1993) notes that the tolerance level for pain can be influenced by a large number of factors, both positive and negative. The threshold for pain tolerance (or perhaps intolerance) may be influenced by any of the following:

- perception of the cause of pain
- uncertainty regarding the cause of pain
- factors associated with the treatment of the underlying disease
- poor communication about the aims of treatment
- other worries and anxieties relating to the context of the pain being experienced
- lack of social support.

It is also suggested (particularly in chronic non-cancer pain) that tolerance levels are reduced the longer pain remains unrelieved. The consequences of unrelieved pain are far-reaching, and as would be expected, have a negative effect on all aspects of a person's life. Additionally, Strang (1998) argues that physical pain provokes emotional, social and existential distress in the patient with cancer. He outlines the negative impact of pain affecting:

- mood
- social activities
- activities of daily living
- sleep
- cognitive functions, and
- the existential domain.

It is also recognised that unrelieved pain can be a precursor to other clinical problems such as depression and severe anxiety. Clearly, if the aim of palliative care nursing is to address the social, emotional and spiritual aspects of suffering, then it is inherent in the nurse's role in managing pain to develop strategies to assess and manage these issues. Interventions for dealing with these, along with guidelines on the pharmacological management, are outlined in the following sections.

Box 2.1   Definitions of pain and related concepts

Definition of pain
'Pain is an unpleasant sensory and emotional experience associated with actual or potential damage'

Pain threshold
'The least experience of pain which a subject can recognise'

Pain tolerance level
'The greatest level of pain which a subject is prepared to tolerate'

Definitions by International Association for the Study of Pain (IASP 1986)

PAIN ASSESSMENT

Pain assessment is the foundation of the nursing management of cancer pain. It is important to identify the presence and severity of pain and the effect of the pain on the individual. Nurses, by virtue of the time they spend with patients, and their role in administering analgesia, have a pivotal role to play in this assessment. However, it must be remembered that pain assessment is a multidisciplinary responsibility and must go 'hand in hand' with a thorough medical examination and investigations into the possible causes of pain.

Pain assessment does not stop with the identification of pain, but needs to be ongoing throughout any treatment – failure to do this results in the under-treatment (and sometimes over-treatment) of a patient in pain. Although pain assessments have their place in assessment (discussed later) they do not replace the need for a nurse to obtain a detailed 'picture', through empathic communication, of the patient's experience.

Steps in pain assessment

The following guidance on pain assessment is broken down into the following three steps.

1. Obtaining 'the pain story'
2. Assessment of the physical component of the pain, including:
   a. Initial assessment
   b. On-going assessment
3. Assessment of the non-physical aspects of pain.

Step 1: The pain story

The initial assessment should be performed when a patient first presents with pain or develops a new pain.

The first step is to build a detailed picture of the patient's experience – it can be helpful to think of this as getting the 'pain story' (see Box 2.2). This assessment should be performed when a patient first presents with pain or develops a new pain. Encouraging a patient to tell their

---

Box 2.2 The 'pain story'

What, if anything, do they think is causing the pain?

When did they first notice this pain?

What else was happening at this time? (i.e. had their drugs been altered, had they recently had any treatment for the underlying illness, etc.)

Has the pain remained constant since they noticed it or is it getting worse?

'pain story' gives clues to the cause of pain and the effect of previous treatment.

Step 2: Assessment of the physical component of the pain

This step consists of detailing the physical signs and symptoms of the current pain. Assessing the physical component of the pain is something that is not limited to nursing practice but can be done equally by medical staff – good interdisciplinary communication is necessary to prevent the patient being subjected to a duplicated pain assessment!

The assessments of the physical components of pain are covered in well-designed pain assessment tools and charts and usually include the following two areas.

Initial assessment This includes determining the following:

- Site or sites of the pain – patients with cancer often have more than one site of pain (Twycross et al 1996).
- Pattern of the pain – is the pain worse at any time of the day or night?
- Aggravating factors – does movement or position affect the pain?
- Relieving factors – concentrating on previous medications or interventions.
- The patient's description of the pain – what does the pain feel like? (i.e. aching, dull, shooting, burning, etc.).

On-going assessment After the above has been performed it is necessary to formally determine the response to treatment. There is still good evidence that nurses continue to underestimate pain (McCaffery & Ferrell 1997), and therefore

where patients should be involved in any assessment. This can be done by asking them to complete a pain assessment tool or by directly questioning them about the following:

The severity of the pain   Although this can be done by simply inquiring about whether the pain is better or worse, it does not provide enough information on which to base future treatment strategies. In an effort to be consistent, it is recommended that a rating scale is used (i.e. 0–10 numerical scale or verbal rating scale, discussed in more detail in Part 2 of this chapter). For patients with multiple pains it is necessary to rate each pain separately. This is more easily achieved using a body chart, to clearly illustrate, with the patient, which pain is being rated.

Response to treatment   One of the most neglected aspects in pain assessment relates to'treatment response. Failure to do this results in the administration of ineffective drugs and at worst increases distress through unwarranted side effects. This is particularly problematic in the case of opioids, when rapid escalation of the dose, without attention to assessment of effectiveness, results in patients experiencing sedation, hallucinations and myoclonic jerks (muscle twitching). This is discussed in more detail in the management of pain in Part 2 of this chapter. When a patient has started taking a new analgesic it is important to determine if this is being effective. As different types of pain (i.e. bone pain, nerve pain) are unlikely to respond equally to the same analgesic drug (i.e. morphine), each pain should be assessed independently. To achieve this, the effectiveness of the analgesic administered must be evaluated by asking the patient to rate the severity of their pain(s) at a time when you expect the drug to have reached its maximum potential benefit. If the patient still reports pain, answers to the following questions need to be determined:

- Has there been any improvement in the patient's rating of the severity of the pain?
- If the analgesic helps, how long does the benefit last?

The answers to these questions will determine whether to modify or change the analgesic regimen (see section on the pharmacological management of cancer pain)

Step 3: Assessment of the non-physical aspects of pain

In addition to the assessment of the above physiological aspects, assessment must cover the effects of the pain on other areas of the patient's life.

It is well documented that unrelieved pain is strongly associated with feelings of anxiety, depression and uncertainty (Strang 1998). Moreover, Arathuzich (1991) showed that in a sample of breast cancer patients in pain, over 50% experienced difficulties with daily activities, disrupted sleep, dependency and helplessness, which contributed to spiritual distress. Clearly, successful pain management requires attention to these issues, and needs to start with assessment.

There is no simple formula to do this, but good communication and assessment skills are a starting point. Often active listening and empathy is enough to help alleviate the distress related to these issues. Although not suitable for every

---

Box 2.3   Assessment of non-physical aspects of pain

Anxiety (about the meaning of the pain)	Helplessness and depression
Do you worry about the possible cause of the pain?	Are you able to sleep at night?
Do you worry about what is going to happen in the future?	Are you able to concentrate?
Do you get a frightened feeling as if something awful is about to happen?	Do you find it difficult to make decisions?
	Are you able to enjoy the things you normally enjoy?
Anxiety (about the treatment of the pain)	**Social worries**
Are you concerned about the treatment of the pain?	Is the pain stopping you doing the things you like to do?
Do you worry about having to take the pain killers?	How is your family managing at home?
	Do you have any money worries?

patient and situation, the probes highlighted in Box 2.3 can be a good starting point in the assessment of these difficulties.

Pain assessment tools

Pain assessment tools are needed primarily for the following reasons:

1. To encourage patient involvement.
2. To provide an accurate and reliable measure of the person's pain over a period of time (i.e. when new interventions are introduced).
3. To provide consistent and accurate record of the patient's pain experience amongst the health care team.

Although it may be possible to perform a good assessment (based on the previous discussion) without an assessment tool, it is unlikely that this will be consistently communicated and sustained over any period of time.

Even though pain assessment tools have been advocated for over a decade (Walker et al 1987, Latham 1990), good evidence remains that they still do not feature in the routine nursing care of patients with pain (Clarke et al 1996). Moreover, often when assessment tools are used, they do not inform subsequent pain management strategies (Carr 1997).

Promoting comfort should be the foundation of nursing practice, and pain assessment is pivotal in the drive to alleviate pain and distress. Without a formalised approach to pain assessment it is doubtful that good pain management can be sustained.

There are many good published examples of pain assessment tools. The core components of the pain assessment tool for patients with chronic/cancer pain should include:

- a body chart – to illustrate multiple pains
- a method of rating the severity of pain
- an area to detail aggravating and relieving factors – particularly whether the pain is worse on movement (incident pain)
- the diurnal variation of pain – noting if pain is worse during the night
- the patient's description of the pain.

The clinical specialty governs the choice of the pain assessment tool. A diary may be more feasible for patients to use in the community (de Wit et al 1999), compared with a detailed chart (which may be appropriate for hospital use – see Fig. 2.1). Where possible, the pain assessment tool needs to be valid and reliable in the population and setting it is intended for. However, as valid and reliable pain assessment tools are not available for every setting, a certain degree of compromise is needed (Part 2 of this chapter discusses the area of pain measurement in more detail). If in doubt, contacting a pain management or palliative care specialist is recommended.

Also, Figure 2.2 gives an example of a pain assessment tool incorporated into an existing BP chart, a necessary compromise to limit paperwork!

THE PHARMACOLOGICAL MANAGEMENT OF CANCER PAIN

Managing cancer pain was the subject of the World Health Organization Working Party in 1996 and their subsequent guidance is the basis for the following paragraphs on the drug management of cancer pain (WHO 1996).

Drug treatment remains the main approach to managing cancer pain and includes a detailed assessment and adherence to the following three principles (WHO 1996).

By mouth

Where possible analgesics should be given by the oral route – it is a common misconception amongst health care staff that systemic routes (intravenous, intramuscular, subcutaneous) of the equivalent oral dose are more efficacious in relieving pain. Systemic routes should be reserved for situations where the patient is unable to take oral medications or when there are doubts about drug absorption in the gastrointestinal tract.

By the clock

Analgesics should be given by the clock (at fixed times) and not on an ad-hoc, or prn (as required),

INITIAL PAIN ASSESSMENT

With patient's help detail area of **each** pain on the body chart below:

Please label **each** pain in the body chart opposite (A, B, C...). Then ask the patient to rate the severity of each pain on the 0–10 scale and record it in the table below.

No pain 0 1 2 3 4 5 6 7 8 9 10 **Worst pain imaginable**

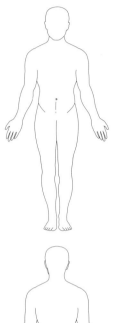

Pain	Severity
A	
B	
C	
D	

Duration of pain

<2 weeks ☐
2–4 weeks ☐
1–2 months ☐
3–6 months ☐
>6 months ☐

Patient's description of pain

What makes the pain worse ?

Does anything help the pain ?

Radiotherapy

Week beginning _____

_____

_____

_____

_____

NB
Any area being irradiated to be
indicated in red on the body chart

Radiotherapy
Commencement date: _____
Dose: _____
Machine: _____
Telephone extension: _____

Figure 2.1   Initial pain assessment.

Western General Hospital NHS Trust Chronic Pain Assessment and Observation Chart

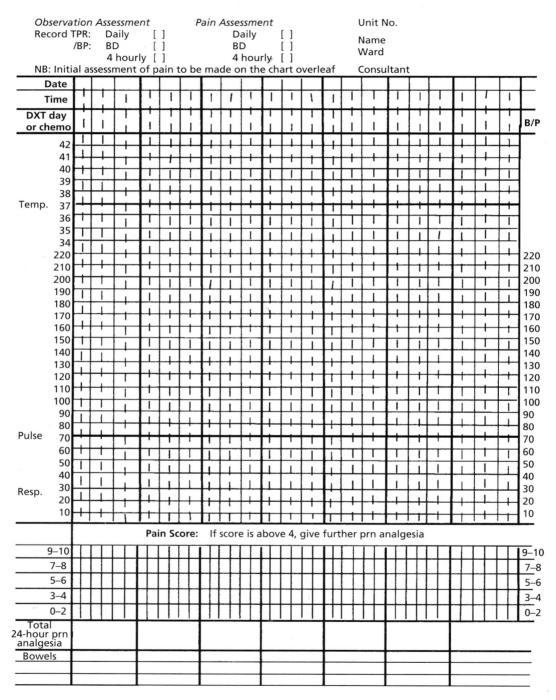

Figure 2.2 Chronic pain assessment and observation chart. (From Western General Hospitals NHS Trust, Edinburgh, with permission.)

The following information details the general principles and guidelines useful in the choice of analgesics for pain in patients with advanced cancer. It is essential that before any analgesics are chosen a detailed assessment of the patient's pain is performed. This must include details on the exact site of the pain; the possible cause of the pain; the type of pain; and its severity.

The World Health Organization recommends that to achieve optimum pain relief analgesia must be given as follows:

- by the mouth
- by the clock (regularly and not on a prn basis)
- by the ladder (see below).

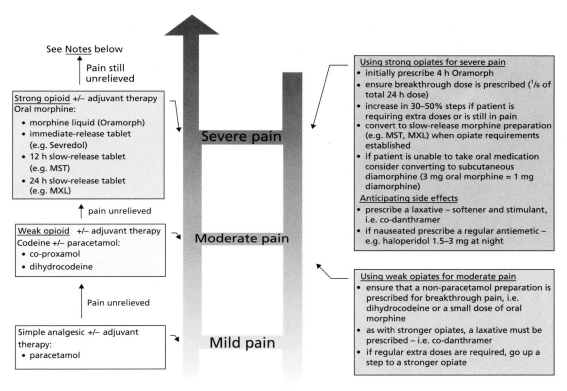

Notes:
1. Pain unrelieved despite strong opioids.

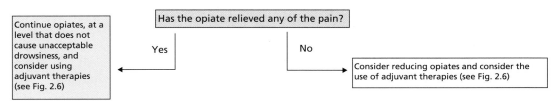

2. For further information on the use of more specific analgesics, i.e. fentanyl (Durogesic) patches or tramadol (Zydol) please contact the Palliative Care Team.

Figure 2.3 Guidelines on the use of analgesics for the patient with advanced cancer. (From Western General Hospitals NHS Trust, Edinburgh, with permission.)

basis. The dose of the analgesic must be titrated against the patient's pain until either a ceiling dose is reached (the maximum recommended dose of the drug), or until the pain is effectively relieved, or until the patient begins to experience intolerable side effects. Extra (prn) doses should be given as required, *in addition* to the fixed intervals doses.

By the ladder

The principles of the analgesic ladder are key features of pain management in palliative care. Analgesics should be prescribed and administered according to both the severity of the pain and the response to the drug(s) prescribed (see Fig. 2.3). These are outlined below.

Step 1: mild pain

Step 1 of the ladder is appropriate for patients with mild pain and involves the use of a non-opioid analgesic such as paracetamol or a non-steroidal anti-inflammatory. If this fails to alleviate the pain (when given 'by the clock'), the prescribing of analgesics should be guided by step 2.

Step 2: moderate pain

This step should be used to treat pain that is mild to moderate or when step 1 has been unsuccessful. There are numerous step 2 analgesics, with most of these drugs containing codeine or similar preparations (i.e. dihydrocodeine). Step 2 analgesics are weak opioids and to be effective should have at least 30 mg of codeine per tablet/capsule. Not all pains respond completely to opioids, and in such instances a non-opioid should be co-prescribed.

Step 3: moderate/severe pain

Drugs in step 3 are those most commonly associated with cancer pain management (frequently morphine in the UK). These drugs are associated with misconceptions surrounding their appropriate use. The choice of a strong opioid should

be governed by the severity of the pain (as reported by the patient) and/or failure of step 2 of the ladder.

The effective dose is whatever relieves the pain and the dose must be gradually increased, until either pain relief is achieved or side effects become problematic. The presence of side effects (such as drowsiness, hallucinations and muscle twitching) are an indication that the dose has been increased too rapidly and/or that the pain is not completely opioid responsive. The principles of administering strong opioids are the same as in step 2, namely given 'by mouth' and 'by the clock'. An appropriate breakthrough drug (prn) must be prescribed, which is normally approximately one-sixth of the total 24-hour opioid dose. If patients are unable to take oral medication then other strong opioids are given by other routes (e.g. subcutaneous or transdermal).

Some pains do not respond completely to opioids (i.e. bone pain and nerve pain) and therefore co-analgesic drugs may need to be prescribed alongside non-opioid and opioid analgesics. Co-analgesics include steroids, tricyclic antidepressants and antiepileptic drugs – a detailed discussion of these drugs is beyond the scope of this chapter and interested readers should consult other texts (e.g. Twycross 1994). Oncological treatments, particularly radiotherapy for bone pain, should always be considered.

OTHER STRATEGIES TO ENHANCE PAIN MANAGEMENT

Anticipating side effects

Many of the side effects commonly associated with analgesics can be anticipated and managed effectively. Constipation is a side effect of all opioids and can be prevented with regular prescriptions of stimulant and softening laxatives. Nausea is normally a transient side effect of opioids, which settles in most patients within a few days, and can be alleviated with a regular antiemetic. Similarly, transient drowsiness associated with opioids that are titrated gradually against pain usually settles within a short period of time. When possible, other drugs that have sedative side effects should be rationalised when opioids are prescribed. If these symptoms do not settle with appropriate treatment, it may be worth trying a different opioid (see Part 2 of this chapter) – before doing this advice should be sought from local palliative care services.

Managing anxieties and fears

The provision of timely and appropriate information will help to ensure compliance with drug regimens and allay anxieties and misconceptions surrounding drug management. Frequently, particularly with recent media reporting surrounding opioid prescribing in terminal care, patients and their families harbour misconceptions about drug treatments. These misconceptions are almost always unfounded and only increase anxiety and distress for the patient and family.

Addiction

Characterised by a craving for the drug and an overwhelming preoccupation with obtaining it (McCaffery & Ferrell 1997), addiction is perhaps the most common fear and misconception and yet is almost never an issue in clinical practice (WHO 1996). Many patients also worry about developing tolerance to the analgesic properties of opioids, but this is rarely a serious clinical issue. In the small group of patients that develop clinically significant tolerance, this can be managed by changing to a different opioid. There are many good booklets available from cancer charities (i.e. BACUP) and pharmaceutical companies that help in providing clear information for patients.

Reassess and seek advice

Pain management based on a meticulous assessment and a structured approach to administering analgesia (using established guidelines) will achieve effective pain control for the majority of patients. A small minority of patients will sometimes experience intractable pain. In these situations it is first necessary to reassess and evaluate the pain and treatments instigated. The patient may have developed a new pain or the pain is not completely opioid-responsive. Lack of attention to the non-physical manifestations and interventions for these will hamper effective pain management.

NON-PHARMACOLOGICAL STRATEGIES FOR THE MANAGEMENT OF CANCER PAIN

There are a number of strategies available to nurses that have been demonstrated to help alleviate pain associated with cancer. Issues relevant to practice are:

- providing relevant and accurate information to the patient and family
- dealing with common myths and misconceptions about cancer pain management
- maximising compliance with analgesic drug regimens.

Although there is a growing body of literature on other non-pharmacological methods for pain management, they are not included in this section because of contradictory evidence about effectiveness. Part 2 addresses some of these issues in more detail.

Providing relevant and accurate information to the patient and family

The provision of accurate verbal and written material has been shown to improve patients' knowledge of pain and to decrease pain intensity (Walker et al 1987, de Wit et al 1999). The pain management strategies outlined previously may seem straightforward to health care professionals but, for patients and families who are unclear about the aims and purposes of the interventions, it can only exacerbate their anxiety. Some drugs are not expected to provide immediate relief, such as antidepressants for nerve pain. This must be explained.

Patients may worry about not being able to take a variety of drugs being used to establish pain control and need reassurance that these often can be simplified – with slow-release analgesic preparations. When good pain control is achieved, the drug regimen should be simplified

Drug Discharge Sheet

Name. . . . .

Name and dose of drug	Purpose	Number of tablets – amount			

Figure 2.4 Drug discharge sheet. (From Western General Hospitals NHS Trust, Edinburgh, with permission.)

and rationalised to avoid confusion about dose intervals and number of drugs to take. Compliance can also be improved by consistent communication; it is good practice to write the drug regimen on paper for patients and families. This should include clear instructions of:

- the drug name (as on the bottle!)
- the purpose of the drug
- the dosage and interval to be taken.

Many pharmacy departments have specific guidelines and existing resources for providing written information to patients. If not, a generic chart is outlined in Figure 2.4.

Dealing with common myths and misconceptions about cancer pain management

Patients and families often have anxieties about the drug management of pain – particularly morphine (Thomason et al 1998). It is important that health care workers are clear about their beliefs and values regarding cancer pain management, before attempting to address patient

---

Box 2.4 Addiction, tolerance and physical dependence

Addiction: craving for the drug and an overall preoccupation with obtaining it.

Tolerance: characterised by decreased efficacy and duration of action with each repeated dose.

Neither tolerance nor addiction is a clinical problem for patients receiving opioids for cancer pain.

Physical dependence: characterised by withdrawal symptoms if the drug is suddenly stopped.

Withdrawal symptoms may arise if the opioid is suddenly stopped – can be avoided by gradual reduction in 25% steps.

Adapted from WHO (1996) *Cancer Pain Relief*. World Health Organization, Geneva.

concerns. Although McCaffery & Ferrell (1997) and Elliott et al (1995), in the United States, have indicated that beliefs about addiction are less prevalent in nursing and medical staff than in previous years, there are still common misconceptions about the related concepts of tolerance and physical dependence (see Box 2.4 for definitions).

Addiction in settings where pain relief is the primary aim is not an issue. A large survey of 12 000 patients on strong opiates, postoperatively, revealed possible problems with addiction in only four patients (Porter & Jick 1980).

Tolerance to opioids is a related but more prevalent misconception amongst patients and health care workers (Elliott et al 1995, Thomason et al 1998). This is not surprising given conflicting views presented in the literature and inaccurate 'media hype' concerning opioid use in terminal care. McCaffery & Ferrell (1997) describe tolerance as being a potential problem for up to 75% of patients on opioids for longer than 3 months. However, it is unclear what evidence this assumption is based on – patients with progressive illnesses are as likely to need increases in analgesia due to increasing disease progression. This view is supported by Elliott et al (1995) who state:

clinically relevant tolerance rarely develops to the analgesic effect of morphine.

Nevertheless it is clear that a few patients develop tolerance, particularly those with unrelieved nerve pain. Strategies for managing tolerance do exist and are outlined in Part 2 of this chapter.

Nurses involved in administering opioids to patients for the first time need to address these misconceptions. Failure to do this may compound anxieties and reduce compliance. The probes, outlined in Box 2.2, are a good starting point. Additionally, a short screening tool has been designed (for the American population) that may be worth further exploration for use in the clinical setting (Ward et al 1993).

CONCLUSION

Although managing cancer pain necessarily involves structured drug interventions, nurses must consider the person behind the pain, including issues surrounding the meaning of pain, the person's social life and the impact of pain on emotional well-being.

Although such an integrated and holistic approach to pain management will achieve pain relief for the majority, there will always be instances when pain relief is difficult to achieve. For this minority it may be necessary to obtain advice from local specialist palliative care services.

Part 2 of this chapter deals in more detail with some of the issues surrounding the more complex and intractable pains.

PART 2: PAIN MANAGEMENT AT A HIGHER LEVEL OF NURSING PRACTICE

INTRODUCTION

Continuing changes in health care delivery are providing nurses with exciting and challenging opportunities. These have 'increased the skills and decision making capacity required of all practitioners' (UKCC 1999).

This part of the chapter examines and outlines some of the more current clinical issues relevant for nurses working at or toward a 'higher level' in pain management in palliative care.

It is anticipated that readers interested in the following paragraphs will be from a variety of areas and backgrounds, including:

- specialist clinical areas – hospice/palliative care, oncology
- community or hospital specialist palliative care services, and
- nurses keen to expand their knowledge and skills in this area.

It is important to point out that the skills and interventions at a higher level should be practised in the context of the anticipated UKCC guidance (UKCC 1999), according to local practice and policies, and within the multidisciplinary ethos of palliative care. The core principles (outlined in Part 1) will make the biggest impact in alleviating cancer pain. Readers should be competent with these skills before considering the following discussions.

The skills required to practice at a 'higher level' within this area are difficult to articulate (Benner 1984) and will develop through extensive clinical practice and exposure to the more complex issues surrounding cancer pain management. Specialist practice in this field is broader than the following discussions on managing complex pain, and necessarily involves a commitment to developing practice through audit, research and education (Humphris 1994, UKCC 1997). The remit of this chapter limits the discussions to the clinical aspects of higher level practice and will specifically address the following issues:

- assessment of complex pain
- recognising and managing opioid toxicity
- developments in the management of complex pain
- managing anxiety associated with pain and suffering.

For clarity, complex pain is defined as pain that is not easily alleviated by the guidelines set out in Part 1 – based on the WHO guidelines (WHO 1996).

ASSESSMENT OF COMPLEX PAIN

The importance of a thorough and meticulous pain assessment cannot be underestimated. An incomplete assessment may be responsible for a 'seemingly' difficult pain to alleviate. The first step in the nursing management of a complex pain is to go 'back to basics' by reassessing the pain and surrounding issues. In many instances this will provide enough information to manage pain. Nurses working at a higher level may need to obtain the necessary knowledge and skills in the following areas.

Physical examination

A physical examination should always be performed as part of any pain assessment, and must be carried out in conjunction with medical staff. This will give clues to possible causes of pain (i.e. constipation, nerve damage, bone involvement) and will guide treatment. Medical staff experi-

---

> **Box 2.5** Definitions of altered skin sensations common in neuropathic pain
>
> Dysaesthesia: an unpleasant abnormal sensation
> Allodynia: pain due to a stimulus which does not normally evoke pain (i.e. light touch)
> Hyperalgesia: an increased response to a stimulus which is normally painful (i.e. a painful perception lasts longer than expected)
> Hyperpathia: an increased pain response with an increased pain perception
> Adapted from Twycross (1994) and IASP (1986).

enced in palliative care will look for pain syndromes to help identify the aetiology of the pain (i.e. lumbar plexopathy, vertebral syndromes or spinal cord compression) (Portenoy & Lesage 1999).

Nurses may need to perform a physical examination, to obtain clues to the possible causes of the pain. This typically will involve looking for obvious sources of pain (i.e. pressure sores, open wounds, etc.) and an examination by light pressure and touch of areas surrounding the pain.

Many pains that are difficult and complex to manage are neuropathic in origin (discussed later), and commonly exhibit peculiar sensations on the skin innervated by the damaged nerve. These sensations have been usefully defined and classified, and form the basis of diagnosing neuropathic pain (see Box 2.5).

Physical examination around the distribution of the pain may reveal one or more of these problems, and should be documented and reported. The creative use of a pain chart to document these is recommended.

Reassess analgesic response to previous treatments

Patients often receive complex drug therapies – often concurrently! It may be difficult to find out what helps, but detailed questioning about the pain and the effectiveness of current and previous interventions is essential for planning future treatments. In the case of opioids it is always beneficial to inquire whether an immediate opioid preparation helps (almost always some benefit from opioids is derived). If at all possible, patients should be asked to rate the severity of their pain following administration of an analgesic (on a numerical or verbal descriptive scale – see Fig. 2.1).

Assessment of other related physical and non-physical problems

Pain does not exist in isolation from the whole person, and as mentioned, the impact of other possible sources of distress must be considered within any assessment. Patients with life-threatening and progressive diseases experience many symptoms and problems that will have a direct bearing on their experience of pain. These problems may be attributed to the global distress and suffering experienced in the context of their illness or related to problems associated with the treatment of the pain.

Pain as a component of suffering

In Part 1 of this chapter the concept of pain thresholds and tolerance were outlined, and these principles remain important in considering the assessment of complex pain. Saunders (1967), using a model called 'total pain', highlighted the many areas of potential suffering that influence pain perception. This model is widely recognised as important for conceptualising the plight of suffering in terminally ill patients (see Fig. 2.5). Similarly, a paper by Cassel (1982) highlights that pain is experienced by the whole person, is linked to suffering and is intensely personal and different between individuals. Any assessment must reflect the complexity of pain and its link with suffering.

In specialist palliative care, it is accepted practice that assessment should be 'problem based', from the patients' perspective, enabling discussion of *their* most pertinent worries and

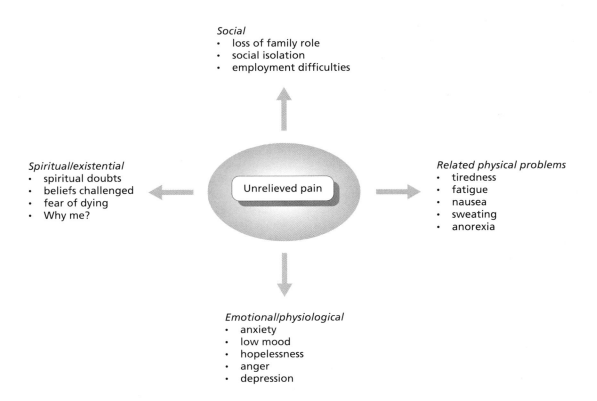

Figure 2.5   The multifaceted nature of pain in palliative care.

difficulties. A problem-based assessment will give clues to other treatable causes of distress and enables support to be focused on areas of difficulties identified by the patient. A problem-based assessment simply involves asking a patient: 'What are your main worries or problems?'. This assessment strategy often highlights that pain, although often severe, is not the main problem. Subsequent attention and support that is directed towards the main problem might help reduce pain perception.

Other clinical problems, not always easily articulated by the patient and family, such as uncertainty, anxiety and depression, may affect pain perception and therefore must be considered in the assessment of complex pain problems.

Assessing side effects – opioid toxicity

The majority of patients can achieve good pain control, and suffer few side effects. Analgesics for the treatment of pain, particularly opioids, are not without potential problems. Opioids are a major cause of constipation, dry mouth, nausea and transient drowsiness, particularly when these are not anticipated and treated. Tolerance to sedation and nausea/vomiting usually occurs within 1 week; however, dry mouth and constipation invariably persist and require ongoing nursing attention. Many other drugs used as co-analgesics and adjuvants for pain relief have potentially problematic side effects, which if undetected will further compound the misery of a patient with complex pain.

Recently, a better understanding of the pharmacokinetics and neurophysiology of opioids has emerged and is changing how we manage opioid side effects. It is postulated that many of the problems associated with 'opioid toxicity' are due to opioid metabolites (a byproduct of opioid metabolism) causing unacceptable side effects in some individuals. While it seems that a small percentage of patients are very sensitive to these metabolites, more frequently this toxicity is the result of the over-zealous use of opioids for pain that is only partially opioid-responsive. Concurrent physical problems such as renal fail-

ure and/or dehydration can lead to the accumulation of some metabolites (which are primarily excreted by the kidneys).

It is thought that two opioid metabolites (morphine-6-glucuronide and morphine-3-glucuronide) are responsible for some of the problems associated with opioid toxicity. These side effects include cognitive impairment (drowsiness and reduced concentration), nausea/vomiting and, in severe cases, myoclonus (muscle twitching), hallucinations and delirium. It is postulated that severe opioid toxicity may be associated with hyperalgesia and allodynia in neuropathic pain (Dickenson 1994).

Opioid toxicity is a common feature in difficult pain problems and is common in the terminal stage of a person's illness, where either the need for opioids has decreased and/or they have developed renal failure or dehydration. In some patients this can lead to the vicious cycle described by O'Neill & Fallon (1998) where opioid toxicity is interpreted as pain, resulting in increased opioids and sedation and leading to further distress from symptoms of toxicity. It is important that nurses learn to recognise these scenarios for which the management is discussed in a later section.

Involve family/carer(s) in the assessment

It is good practice to involve the family in all aspects of palliative care provision, enabling more detailed account of the background to the patient's experiences to be gained. The family may have concerns and worries about the pain and its treatment. A close family member may confirm any worries about issues such as compliance and confusion over drug regimens. Failure to involve and support relatives is postulated by Meittinen et al (1998) as one indicator of the probability of inappropriate pain control.

THE MANAGEMENT OF COMPLEX PAIN

The management of complex pain requires the full attention of the multidisciplinary team. Although many interventions revolve around drug therapies, this should not be at the expense of other non-pharmacological methods. The following discussions presume that the approaches covered in Part 1 have been exhausted.

Pharmacological interventions

Complex pains are almost always opioid-responsive but the degree of relief obtained may vary considerably between individuals. As in some cases it is undesirable side effects that limit the use of appropriate doses of opioids, the following questions need to be explored:

1. Does the opioid relieve the pain but side effects prevent required increase in the opioid?
2. Is the pain only partially relieved by the opioid despite incremental increases in the dose?

Rapid escalation of the opioid in the presence of side effects and/or the absence of an analgesic response will produce the symptoms of opioid toxicity previously described. Managing opioid toxicity is directed at treating the causes and palliating side effects. This involves:

- reducing the opioids gradually
- treating dehydration and reversible causes of renal failure
- stopping or reducing other drugs which may be contributing to the problem
- treating delirium and hallucinations (with drugs such as haloperidol/droperidol).

If pain remains a problem and side effects prevent increases in the dose, trying a different strong opioid is indicated.

Alternative opioids

A better understanding of opioid side effects (including the role of morphine metabolites) has enabled the development of a clearer strategy in the management of pain that is opioid-responsive but limited by side effects. These strategies focus on changing to a different opioid ('opioid switching' or 'rotation') – with the hope that the patient will experience fewer side effects and therefore tolerate a higher dose (Olson & Sjogren 1996). For many years morphine and diamorphine have been the only strong opioids used in palliative and terminal care, but alternatives enable opioid 'switching' to be a realistic option. These opioids include:

- hydromorphone
- fentanyl
- oxycodone
- methadone.

Each of these opioids has different properties and differing potencies compared with morphine. Conversion ratios from one opioid to another need to be treated with caution, as considerable variability exists between individuals. Switching opioids requires careful monitoring and supervision.

Pain poorly responsive to opioids

Complex pain that is not alleviated by opioids is treated, in the first instance, by adjuvant analgesics. The choice of drug is dependent on the cause of the pain, as illustrated in Figure 2.6. A discussion of all of these is beyond the scope of the chapter and therefore readers are encouraged to consult other authoritative texts (Twycross 1994). When appropriate it may be necessary to treat the cause of the pain. This may involve radiotherapy, chemotherapy and, in some instances, surgery. The possible benefits of these treatments for each individual must be balanced against risks and possible side effects.

As pain from nerve damage disproportionately represents causes of complex pain, the following discussion will outline some of the available treatment options.

Neuropathic pain

Pain due to nerve damage (neuropathic pain) can arise from a multitude of factors and in the case of cancer pain may be tumour-related or treatment-related. There are a wide variety of

The choice of co-analgesic depends on the likely cause of the pain, making a detailed reassessment of the patient's pain crucial. Below are some of the common pains that do not always respond totally to the use of opioids, and suggestions for their management.

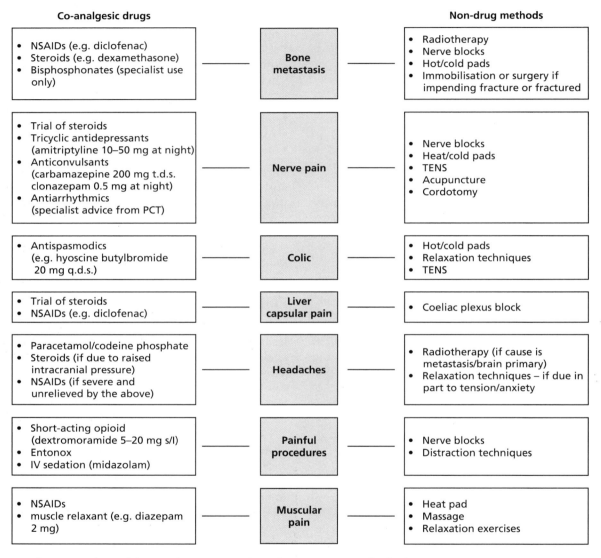

Co-analgesic drugs		Non-drug methods
• NSAIDs (e.g. diclofenac) • Steroids (e.g. dexamethasone) • Bisphosphonates (specialist use only)	**Bone metastasis**	• Radiotherapy • Nerve blocks • Hot/cold pads • Immobilisation or surgery if impending fracture or fractured
• Trial of steroids • Tricyclic antidepressants (amitriptyline 10–50 mg at night) • Anticonvulsants (carbamazepine 200 mg t.d.s. clonazepam 0.5 mg at night) • Antiarrhythmics (specialist advice from PCT)	**Nerve pain**	• Nerve blocks • Heat/cold pads • TENS • Acupuncture • Cordotomy
• Antispasmodics (e.g. hyoscine butylbromide 20 mg q.d.s.)	**Colic**	• Hot/cold pads • Relaxation techniques • TENS
• Trial of steroids • NSAIDs (e.g. diclofenac)	**Liver capsular pain**	• Coeliac plexus block
• Paracetamol/codeine phosphate • Steroids (if due to raised intracranial pressure) • NSAIDs (if severe and unrelieved by the above)	**Headaches**	• Radiotherapy (if cause is metastasis/brain primary) • Relaxation techniques – if due in part to tension/anxiety
• Short-acting opioid (dextromoramide 5–20 mg s/l) • Entonox • IV sedation (midazolam)	**Painful procedures**	• Nerve blocks • Distraction techniques
• NSAIDs • muscle relaxant (e.g. diazepam 2 mg)	**Muscular pain**	• Heat pad • Massage • Relaxation exercises

Note: These are only guidelines – please contact the Palliative Care Team for further advice.

Figure 2.6 Adjuvant therapies and co-analgesics for pain management. (From Western General Hospitals NHS Trust, Edinburgh, with permission.)

other causes of neuropathic pain not related to cancer – often evident in chronic pain syndromes (i.e. phantom limb pain, post-stroke pain or diabetic peripheral neuropathy).

The first step in managing neuropathic pain in palliative care is to apply the previously outlined analgesic ladder. In some instances neuropathic pain may be very opioid-responsive, but in other cases strategies warrant the use of co-analgesics (see Fig. 2.6). Numerous co-analgesics are reported to help nerve pain, but the evidence in cancer pain is sparse. The following drug classes are those with evidence of effectiveness in the chronic pain (non-cancer) population or from clinical consensus (not proven in clinical trials):

- anticonvulsant drugs (McQuay et al 1995)
- tricyclic antidepressants (McQuay & Moore 1997)
- steroids.

If these co-analgesics, along with opioids, do not produce adequate analgesia, other drug and non-drug methods must be considered.

There is growing interest in drugs that dampen down excitatory neural activity, postulated to be one of the causes of neuropathic pain (Ventafridda et al 1996). This phenomenon of abnormal neural activity in the spinal cord is commonly called *wind-up*, and may occur in the absence of a painful stimulus. It has been shown (in animal models) that certain drugs block the *N*-methyl-D-aspartate (NMDA) receptor thought to be important in the development of 'wind-up' (Dickenson 1994). The common drugs used for this purpose include ketamine and methadone:

- ketamine does not have analgesic properties per se but can alleviate neuropathic pain by blocking NMDA receptors in the spinal cord (Mercadante 1996)
- methadone, a strong opioid, has a potential to block this receptor (Morley & Makin 1998).

As with the discussion of alternative opioids, use of these drugs requires a specialist knowledge and experience and careful monitoring of potential side effects is necessary.

Finally, neuropathic pain and other complex pains of different origin may not always be completely amenable to drug treatment and therefore non-drug interventions may be necessary (see Fig. 2.6). The complexity and difficulties in managing these pains highlight the need for good links with other disciplines, including palliative medicine, oncology and chronic pain management.

NON-PHARMACOLOGICAL MANAGEMENT OF DISTRESS ASSOCIATED WITH PAIN

The importance of conceptualising pain as a multifaceted concept, as outlined in Figure 2.5, has been discussed previously. In recognising the multifaceted experience of pain in palliative care, attention to non-physical distress needs intervention alongside the management of the physical component of the pain. For this to occur it is necessary for open and honest communication to take place in all stages of palliative care provision. Such communication must constantly assess for possible non-physical causes of distress that impact on the patient's pain perception. The possible causes of such distress have been thoroughly documented in the palliative care literature (Saunders 1967, Cassel 1982) and in many instances can be addressed through good communication and active steps to support the patient and family during their illness. Nurses working at a higher level of clinical practice need to use well-developed communication skills to ensure that patients are constantly informed and involved in the decision-making process that is required to manage pain. Encouraging patients who are able to take an active role in the management of their pain has been clearly demonstrated to produce positive outcomes (de Wit et al 1995) and is particularly important when pain is not easily alleviated by the more straightforward strategies outlined in Part 1 of this chapter. Involving patients and families in the management of their pain is not always easy, as their decisions may not always be what we would choose on their behalf. Health care professionals need to remain flexible and open minded in their willingness to engage individuals in their care, while at the same time ensuring that they have correct and accurate information to enable informed decision making.

For some patients, the active role that they adopt may involve trying non-pharmacological interventions that are not traditionally associated with the medical management of pain in palliative care. These may include interventions such as:

- imagery
- music therapy/art therapy
- acupuncture
- TENS
- aromatherapy
- relaxation.

While there may be little scientific evidence of the benefits of some of these therapies for pain management in palliative care (Sindhu 1996), patients who choose to try these therapies should be supported – at the very least because it encourages them to take an active role in the management of their pain.

It is necessary to ensure that these therapies are practised safely and are not contraindicated with other treatments. Any nurses offering such interventions must ensure that they operate within professional guidelines (UKCC 1997) and according to local policies.

The role of relaxation techniques in cancer pain management deserves further investigation and discussion. Relaxation techniques are commonly used within chronic pain management programmes and there is emerging evidence that some patients in the palliative care population will benefit from some form of relaxation training (Syrjala & Donaldson 1995). More research is needed to demonstrate its effectiveness (Wallace 1997), in particular to determine which groups will derive the most benefit. The relationship between pain and anxiety is suggested by Montes-Sandoral (1999) to be reciprocal and interconnected at both the physical and non-physical level. Although this relationship is not fully understood, it is clear that for some individuals relaxation therapies will reduce pain. Nurses working at a higher level in palliative care must develop the skills needed to offer relaxation training to patients. Teaching patients relaxation invariably opens up opportunities to discuss other worries and anxieties that they may be experiencing. There are many forms of relaxation therapies, but whatever is offered must be simple and practical in the clinical area it is being used in. Most community and hospital services have liaison psychiatry services that will be able to advise and teach nurses practical relaxation techniques.

CONCLUSION

Part 2 of this chapter aimed to introduce readers to some of the newer developments in pain management in palliative care and outline the importance of good communication for patients and their families. Evidence of the effectiveness of some interventions (such as relaxation) exists; there is a need for nurses practising at a higher level to engage in further research to evaluate their effectiveness and develop methods of introducing them into clinical practice. Nurses must participate and initiate programmes of clinical audit to determine what areas within their practice need improvement (see Farrer 1999 for a full discussion of research and audit in palliative care nursing).

Additionally, Part 2 of this chapter has discussed some of the developments in cancer pain management, in particular in relation to neuropathic pain. While our understanding of neuropathic pain is increasing, this is a rapidly evolving area which will hopefully lead to improved treatments.

Although current developments in the treatment of intractable cancer pain are important, it must be remembered that the core principles outlined in Part 1 of this chapter will bring the most benefit to the majority of patients. The responsibility of nurses working at a higher level of practice must extend beyond the application of the more specialist pain management strategies, to ensuring through educational initiatives that all colleagues within the multidisciplinary team are conversant with the core principles of cancer pain management.

REFERENCES

Arathuzich D 1991 Pain experience for metastatic breast cancer patients. Cancer Nursing 14: 41–48

Benner P 1984 From novice to expert: excellence and power in clinical nursing practice. Addison Wesley, London

Bonica J J 1990 Cancer pain: current status and future needs: In: Bonica J J (ed) The management of pain. Lea & Febiger, Philadelphia

Bowsher D 1993 Pain management in nursing: In: Bowsher D, Carroll C (eds) Pain management and nursing care. Butterworth Heinemann, Oxford

Carr E C J 1997 Evaluating the use of a pain assessment tool and care plan: a pilot study. Journal of Advanced Nursing 26: 1073–1079

Cassel E J 1982 The nature of suffering and the goals of medicine. The New England Journal of Medicine 306(11): 639–645

Clarke E B, French B, Bilodeau M L, Caapasso V C, Edwards A, Empoliti J 1996 Pain management, knowledge, attitudes and clinical practice: the impact of nurses' characteristics and education. Journal of Pain and Symptom Management 11(1): 18–31

Cleeland C S, Gonin R et al 1994 Pain and its treatment in outpatients with metastatic cancer. New England Journal of Medicine 330(9): 592–596

de Wit R, van Dam F S, van Buuren A et al 1995 Pain counselling for chronic cancer pain patients: a nursing intervention study (meeting abstract). 7th International Symposium on Supportive Care in Cancer, September

de Wit R, van Dam F, Hanneman M et al 1999 Evaluation of the use of a pain diary in chronic cancer pain patients at home. Pain 79(1): 89–99

Dickenson A H 1994 Neurophysiology of opioid poorly responsive pain: In: Hanks G W (ed.) Palliative medicine: problem areas in pain and symptom management. CSHL Press, New York, p. 21

Elliott B A, Murray D M, Elliott T E et al 1995 Physicians' knowledge and attitudes about cancer pain management: a survey from the Minnesota Cancer Pain Management Project. Journal of Pain and Symptom Management 19(7): 494–504

Farrer K 1999 Research and audit: demonstrating quality. In: Lugton J, Kindlen M (eds) Palliative care: the nursing role. Churchill Livingstone, Edinburgh

Grond S, Zech D, Diefenbach C, Radbruch L, Lehmann K A 1996 Assessment of cancer pain: a prospective evaluation in 2266 cancer patients referred to a pain service. Pain 64(1): 107–114

Hanks G W, Forbes K 1997 Opioid responsiveness. Acta Anaesthesiologica Scandinavica 41(1 Pt 2): 154–158

Humphris D 1994 The clinical nurse specialist – issues in practice. Macmillan, Basingstoke

IASP 1986 Subcommittee on taxonomy. Pain (Suppl) 3: 216–221

Latham J 1990 Pain control. Austin Cornish, London

McCaffery M, Ferrell B R 1997 Nurses' knowledge of pain assessment and management: how much progress have we made? Journal of Pain and Symptom Management 14(3): 175–188

McQuay H C, Moore A 1997 Bibliography and systematic reviews in cancer pain: a report to the NHS National Cancer Research and Development Programme, Oxford

McQuay H, Carroll D, Jadad A R, Wiffen P, Moore A 1995 Anticonvulsant drugs for management of pain: a systematic review. British Medical Journal 311(21 October 1995): 1047–1052

Meittinen T, Tilvis R, Karppi P, Arve S 1998 Why is pain relief of dying patients often unsuccessful? The relatives' perspectives. Palliative Medicine 12(6): 429–453

Mercadante S 1996 Ketamine in cancer pain: an update. Palliative Medicine 10: 225–230

Montes-Sandoval L 1999 An analysis of the concept of pain. Journal of Advanced Nursing 29(4): 935–941

Morley J S, Makin M K 1998 The use of methadone in cancer pain poorly responsive to other opioids. Pain Reviews 5: 51–58

Olson A K, Sjogren P 1996 Neurotoxic effects of opioids. European Journal of Palliative Care 3(4): 139–142

O'Neill B, Fallon M F 1998 Principles of palliative care and pain control: In: O'Neill B, Fallon M F (eds) ABS of palliative care. BMJ Books, London

Paice J P, Toy C, Shott S 1998 Barriers to cancer pain relief: fear of tolerance and addiction. Journal of Pain and Symptom Management 16(1): 1–9

Portenoy R L, Lesage P 1999 Management of cancer pain. Lancet 353: 1695–1700

Porter J, Jick H 1980 Addiction rare in patients treated with narcotics. New England Journal of Medicine 302: 123

Saunders C M 1967 The management of terminal illness. Hospital Medicine Publications, London

Sindhu F 1996 Are non-pharmacological nursing interventions for the management of pain effective? – a meta-analysis. Journal of Advanced Nursing 24: 1152–1159

Strang P 1998 Cancer pain – a provoker of emotional, social and existential distress. Acta Oncologica 37(7/8): 641–644

Syrjala K L, Donaldson G W 1995 Relaxation and imagery and cognitive behaviour training reduce pain during cancer treatment: a controlled trial. Pain 63: 189–198

Thomason T E, McCune J S, Bernard S A, Winer E P, Tremont S, Lindley C M 1998 Cancer pain survey: patient-centered issues in control. Journal of Pain and Symptom Management 15(5): 275–284

Twycross R 1994 Pain relief in advanced cancer. Churchill Livingstone, London

Twycross R, Harcourt J, Bergl S 1996 A survey of pain in patients with advanced cancer. Journal of Pain and Symptom Management 12(5): 273–282

UKCC 1997 Prep – the nature of advanced practice. UKCC, London

UKCC 1999 A higher level of practice. UKCC, London

Ventafridda V, Tamburini M, Caraceni A, De Conno F, Naldi F 1987 A validation study of the WHO method for cancer pain relief. Cancer 59(4): 850–856

Ventafridda V, Caraceni A, Sbanotto A 1996 Cancer pain management. Pain Reviews 3(3): 153–179

Walker V A, Dicks B, Webb P 1987 Pain assessment charts in the management of chronic cancer pain. Palliative Medicine 1: 111–116

Wallace K G 1997 Analysis of recent literature concerning relaxation and imagery interventions for cancer pain. Cancer Nursing 20: 87–97

Ward S, Goldberg N, Millar-McCauley V 1993 Patient related barriers to management of cancer pain. Pain 52: 319–324

WHO 1996 Cancer pain relief. World Health Organization, Geneva

3

Assessment of symptoms

Anita Roberts   Adele Bird

INTRODUCTION

Palliative care aims to relieve physical, psychological, social and spiritual symptoms (Bruera et al 1991). The assessment of symptoms and symptom distress is, therefore, a vital aspect of nursing patients with advanced and incurable disease. Symptom management should be guided by a comprehensive assessment that incorporates an understanding of the multidimensional nature of symptoms and quality of life for the individual (Ingham & Portenoy 1996). Symptom control is a major goal within palliative care and, if the success of this goal is to be measured, adequate methods of assessing symptoms and the distress they cause are required (Sutcliffe-Chidgey & Holmes 1996).

SYMPTOMS – A GENERAL DEFINITION

The study of symptoms has been hampered to some degree by a lack of consistency in terminology. A symptom has been defined as 'a subjective indication of a disease, i.e. something perceived by the patient' (Ingham & Portenoy 1996). While a generally accepted definition for 'pain' exists and there has been the development of a taxonomy for the study of this symptom, no such definition has evolved to clarify other symptoms. For example, the measurement of 'fatigue', 'confusion', and even 'breathlessness', is complicated by the absence of specific definitions. Symptom assessment and measurement is dependent on the clarity of meanings attached to descriptions of symptoms given.

PREVALENCE OF SYMPTOMS

Palliative care is no longer exclusively available for patients with cancer. Patients with any life-threatening disease may need palliative care and there is a great diversity in the range of symptoms these patients present with. Studies focusing on the prevalence of symptoms in advanced disease have concentrated on the patient with advanced cancer. Twycross (1997) identifies the following symptoms:

- physical – lack of energy, pain, drowsiness, dry mouth, nausea and anorexia
- psychological – worrying, feeling sad, feeling nervous, difficulty sleeping, feeling irritable and difficulty concentrating.

One of the earliest surveys of symptoms was carried out by Dunlop in 1989. The 10 most prevalent symptoms identified were weakness, dry mouth, anorexia, depression, difficulty in sleeping, pain, swollen legs, nausea, constipation and vomiting. This is comparable to Twycross' list. A further study by Curtis et al (1991) identified the following 10 most common symptoms: pain, weight loss, anorexia, dyspnoea, constipation, early satiety, fatigue, dry mouth, weakness and nausea. All three studies involved interviews with patients on admission to a care facility. The National Council for Hospices and Specialist Palliative Care Services (1998) identifies that patients dying from non-malignant disease have similar symptoms to those with malignant disease, especially in respect of nausea and anorexia.

Assessment is a vital aspect of patient care. It forms the basis for any subsequent intervention. Therefore, the purpose of nursing assessment is to provide an accurate picture of the patient's current position (Crow et al 1995). It is important that nurses, together with other health care professionals, can establish the needs of patients receiving palliative care accurately, so that care can be planned for any physical, social and psy-

chological needs (Tiffany & Webb 1988). In this way, the quality of life for these patients can be optimised.

To achieve this level of assessment, the nurse needs to collect information about the patient's current medical condition and also the patient's beliefs, expectations and understanding of the situation and how he or she is coping with what is happening. This assessment involves two broad areas, the assessment and measurement of specific systems and the assessment process itself. Both these areas will be discussed.

THE PROCESS OF ASSESSMENT

Assessment must be regarded as an ongoing process, with information being gathered during the initial assessment but added to and revised over time. It is not vital that everything is covered in great depth during the initial assessment, but it is useful to ascertain the main problems or concerns of the patient (Maguire 1985). By obtaining an accurate assessment the nurse will have a much clearer picture of what the patient has experienced and therefore have a better understanding of the situation from the patient's perspective.

The quality of assessment can be affected by both health care professionals and by patients. Studies have shown that dying patients can suffer uncontrolled symptoms such as pain, anxiety, depression and anorexia (Hockley et al 1988, Higginson et al 1994). Studies have shown that this happened because these patients had not had their needs assessed adequately. More recently, Heaven & Maguire (1996) found that nurses identified less than 40% of their patients' concerns. Wilkinson (1991) has identified key elements which need to be addressed if a comprehensive initial assessment of the patient is to be obtained (Box 3.1).

It has been suggested that nurses and other health care professionals find it easier to assess physical problems than psychological problems (Wilkinson 1991). Patients may be selective in the concerns they choose to disclose. They appear more likely to disclose concerns relating to the physical aspects of their situation. This is even

---

> **Box 3.1** The key areas of a nursing assessment. (Adapted from Wilkinson 1991)
>
> Introduction to nursing assessment
> Patients' understanding of reason for admission/visit
> Patients' awareness of diagnosis/condition
> Patients' history of present illness
> Patients' history of previous illness
> Physical assessment of patient
> Social/spiritual assessment of patient
> Psychological assessment
> Closure of nursing assessment

more probable if the patient is suffering from anxiety or depression (Heaven & Maguire 1997). Given the incidence of these symptoms in patients receiving palliative care, this has important implications for health care professionals. Health care professionals can improve patients' disclosure of psychological concerns by addressing the way they assess patients (Maguire 1985).

If nurses are to elicit the exact nature of the patients' problems, their perceptions and the impact these are having on the patient, the assessment must concentrate on the current situation and what is expected to happen in the future. It is also important for the nurse to find out about what has happened to the patient previously in order to put their present feeling and emotions into context. This may be important if this is the first time the nurse has met the patient. Marks et al (1991) found that some assessment schedules may not always take the previous health of individual patients into account and suggest that nurses wanting to obtain a subjective assessment may need to pay attention to this area.

If there is very limited time in which to undertake the initial assessment or if the patient is very ill, focusing on the patient's current concerns will provide the most valuable information. If it is possible to adopt a wider focus by exploring not only the current concerns but also the initial symptoms, perceptions and emotions, together with any treatments or interventions the patient might have had, this gives the nurse a much better understanding of the patient's situation. It also allows the nurse to gain a clearer picture of how much the patient understands about the illness and what it means to that individual.

Patients may not disclose their concerns because they feel that the health care professional is too busy to listen, or think that their worries and concerns may be too trivial (Maguire 1985). Consequently, the introduction to the assessment is an important part of the process. The nurse needs to ensure that his or her name and role is known by the patient. This helps to establish trust between the patient and nurse and can encourage the patient to disclose concerns. It is also helpful to give a clear purpose for the interview. In this way it is clear that assessment is not a casual conversation and shows that the nurse is interested in hearing about the patient's concerns. If time is limited, it may be helpful to tell the patient how long the assessment is envisaged to last. This allows the patient to discuss what they feel is important. In an assessment there is a professional agenda and the patient's agenda. Both need to be covered and, if time is limited, care must be taken that one area is not overlooked. It is better to leave the professional agenda to the end of the assessment to ensure that it does not diminish the importance of the patient's agenda.

Nurses and other health care professionals are more confident in their ability to assess physical aspects than psychological aspects of illness. This may be because nurses lack the skills needed to communicate effectively (Macleod Clark 1981, Heaven & Maguire 1996). Other reasons include worries about upsetting the patient, not being able to answer difficult questions, saying the wrong things (Maguire 1985), getting into trouble and upsetting the system (Menzies 1961, Maguire 1985). Some nurses find talking about emotional issues so upsetting that they avoid this area to protect themselves (Menzies 1961, Wilkinson 1991).

In many ways the information that is required to assess a physical problem is equally applicable to assessing psychological concerns (Box 3.2). Studies by (Tait et al 1982, Wilkinson et al 1998) have demonstrated that appropriate training can help to improve nurses' communication skills and confidence.

To encourage patients to disclose psychological concerns, nurses must demonstrate very early in the assessment process that they are equally

---

Box 3.2 Assessment information

Nature of problem
Location
Severity
Frequency
Duration
Aggravating factors
Alleviating factors
Effect on activities of daily living
Effect on patient's mood and morale

---

concerned about the emotional aspects as well as the physical facts (Maguire 1985). This is important because if the assessment focuses only on the physical facts early in the assessment, the patient is less likely to disclose any psychological concerns even if asked. This is because the patient feels that the nurse is more concerned about the physical aspects. To avoid relaying this impression, the nurse should establish what kind of impact the symptoms, treatment and other interventions have had on the patient both physically and emotionally.

When ending the assessment, care must be taken to check that important issues have not been missed. This can be done by summarising what has been said, so that the patient can verify the accuracy and misunderstandings are minimised. The patient should also be encouraged to ask any outstanding questions he or she might have. Once this has been done, the nurse can tell the patient what actions need to be taken and what care or treatment will be given.

ASSESSMENT AND MEASUREMENT OF SPECIFIC SYMPTOMS

As discussed, the optimum approach to symptom assessment and measurement must incorporate both patient ratings and physical phenomena. For example, dyspnoea measurement may be complemented by measurement of oxygen saturation or blood gases. Nausea measurement may be supplemented by assessment of the frequency of vomiting (Bruera et al 1991). Symptoms are multidimensional experiences that may be evaluated in terms of their specific characteristics and impact. The impact of symp-

toms may be described in relation to functioning, i.e. family, social, financial or physical, or in relation to wider concepts such as symptom distress or quality of life (Ingham & Portenoy 1996).

It is important to remember that symptoms usually change over time. The symptom itself may remit or recur, or its characteristics may change. In practice, repeated assessments throughout the course of the patient's care will allow this to be monitored adequately.

The challenge of symptom measurement is to capture relevant symptoms as they evolve using measures that are simple and brief so as not to overburden the patient or carer. Several factors influence changes in symptom prevalence and characteristics, including the disease, availability of treatment, changes in function or psychosocial status. Symptoms described by the patient as severe can have an increasing or decreasing impact on associated distress and quality of life (Ingham & Portenoy 1996).

Rathbone et al (1994) suggest that measurement of quality of life in the patient with advanced disease, such as a patient in a hospice, presents many difficulties because of a natural reluctance to make demands on someone whose physical condition is poor and whose life expectancy is short. When providing palliative care the best quality of life possible should be the goal and some attempt at its assessment could be considered important.

SYMPTOM ASSESSMENT AND MEASUREMENT

Effective care programmes rely on comprehensive symptom assessment. Traditionally, symptom checklists, which have been developed to explore common physical and psychological symptoms in particular disease states, have been used to monitor symptoms. These simple instruments have notable limitations, which include the lack of adequate validation and the inability to address more than one symptom (Ingham & Portenoy 1996). Recent studies (MacAdam & Smith 1987, Rathbone et al 1994) have yielded validated measures that address these limitations. In palliative care units, these tools may focus staff attention on symptom assessment, act as a means of reviewing the quality of patient care and demonstrate potential situation-specific barriers to symptom control.

Validated instruments for symptom assessment

There are a variety of tools available to assess symptoms. These have been developed predominately in oncology to monitor the effects of treatment on patients. The selection of an appropriate instrument in palliative care must address this divide. For example, the goal of assessment may be different. The practicality, applicability, and acceptability of the instrument to palliative care patients must be considered. This includes the impact of the measure on both patient and health care professional. Simple and brief measurement strategies limit patient burden and encourage compliance but the complexities of symptom-related concerns or quality of life cannot be ignored. If the information is salient and would not be assessed otherwise, the increased burden may be warranted (Ingham & Portenoy 1996). Although the overall symptom experience of the patient is multidimensional, it has been demonstrated by de Haes et al (1990) that physical and psychological symptoms can be distinguished empirically.

Instruments for the measurement of multiple symptoms

Several well-validated tools are now available to measure quality of life in cancer in palliative care patients. Examples of common tools are listed below.

Rotterdam Symptom Checklist

The Rotterdam Symptom Checklist (RSCL) is a validated, patient-rated measure that evaluates a range of common symptoms in terms of patient-rated distress. The Rotterdam Symptom Checklist provides quantitative information about global symptom distress and sub-scales that distinguish physical and psychological symptom distress.

Some symptoms that may be common in advanced disease, such as change in taste and appearance, are not evaluated.

The scaling of the RSCL (1–4, none, a little, quite often, very often) appears acceptable. However, Sutcliffe-Chidgey & Holmes (1996) advocate that the addition of a category to mark the presence of a symptom which did not cause distress would be useful in assessing the whole patient.

Symptom Distress Scale

The Symptom Distress Scale is a 13-item, patient-rated scale that evaluates 11 symptoms, nine physical and two psychological, in terms of frequency, intensity or distress. Although it only provides limited information about specific symptoms, it is a valid and useful measure of global symptom distress.

Instruments for the measurement of specific symptoms

Although numerous instruments have been validated for the assessment of some symptoms, such as pain and depression, there is a lack of similar instruments for other symptoms that are prevalent in advanced disease, such as anorexia, dry mouth or alterations in body image. Moreover, those symptom-specific instruments that have been validated have been used in specific populations and this may limit their validity in others. For example, many dyspnoea measurements have been developed in respiratory medicine and cardiology and there is little information specifically derived in an oncology or palliative care setting.

Palliative care or hospice interdisciplinary teams caring for a dying person must assess the needs of that person and rank any problems in order of priority for the patient (MacAdam & Smith 1987). This requires a team approach, as visits by each discipline for assessment purposes may be tiring for the patient. The degree of distress experienced when a symptom is present is unique to every individual (Sutcliffe-Chidgey & Holmes 1996). As symptom distress experienced

4

Promoting comfort for patients with symptoms other than pain

Joanne Atkinson   Alison Virdee

INTRODUCTION

For most patients with progressive disease, uncontrolled symptoms can severely affect quality of life and their family's ability to cope with their illness and subsequent death (Higginson 1997). There are many definitions of palliative care, all of which highlight the need to control symptoms and support the family and carers. These principles and practices are not solely the responsibility of palliative care specialists. Relief of symptoms and support of the patient and the carers should be an integral part of health care. While the palliative care approach should be a general principle for all clinical practice, some patients will require physical, psychological, social and spiritual support from a specialist palliative care service to effectively manage their symptoms.

The overall goal is to relieve suffering with due regard to appearance and self-esteem; to maintain activity, independence and something of a normal life... at home if possible if that is what is wanted. This requires individualised care that takes account of the whole person, their circumstances and their wishes.

Diseases need medicine but human beings who suffer will always need a touch of magic.
(Buckman & Sabbagh 1993)

Patients may experience severe physical symptoms which are most often entwined with their

an agreed plan of care by contributing professionals . . . in which basic principles of treatment are translated into daily practice. Each episode of care can be described, tracked and monitored so that intermediate and final outcomes are measured. Care pathways can be used as a means of outlining the expected and realistic course of that patient's care as well as a way of evaluating that care.

Health professionals need to journey along this pathway of care with the patient and family.

Shared decision making

As previously discussed, decisions about treatments and management should be informed by a range of physical, medical and psychosocial issues. These decisions need to be taken with the patient wherever possible so that the patient is able to make an informed choice, even if that choice is to 'leave it up to the experts'. The patient needs clear information about their illness all along the pathway, with clear goals of treatment (Saunders 1993). The patient and family know how important life satisfaction, social, occupational, family roles, sexuality, mood and ability to function, think and concentrate are to them. All these factors colour the decisions they make about treatment (O'Boyle & Waldron 1997).

Re-evaluation

Symptoms change as disease progresses. Therefore, a constant dialogue with the patient and family is needed to maintain effective symptom management.

Monitoring for side effects, worsening disease and drug interactions, as well as signs that a therapy is no longer needed, will enhance symptom management and the quality of life.

Effect on health professionals

The discomfort felt by patients and their families can evoke intense feelings in health professionals which may profoundly affect the way these patients are cared for and the way in which their problems are approached (Stiefel & Guex 1996). An Australian postal survey in 1995 examining the factors which influence medical practitioners' treatment decisions for palliative care patients, showed that their decisions varied according to individual characteristics of the doctor and not solely the nature of the medical problem (Waddell et al 1996). It can be hard to continue dialogue in the same way with patients whose discomfort does not respond to treatment (Saunders 1993). This may be due to health professionals' need to feel that their efforts are productive. To ensure a consistent approach to managing patients' symptoms, an awareness is needed of the possible effects that the beliefs and attitudes of each health care professional may have (see Box 4.1).

Incidence of symptoms: who has symptoms?

Of 627 600 people who died in the UK in 1994, 25% had cancer (Office of National Statistics 1997). One of the main problems for people

---

Box 4.1 Basic rules of symptom management

Assess and record symptoms through dialogue with patient and family
Have a thorough knowledge of pathophysiology, disease process and other illnesses
Have knowledge of treatment, side effects and time lag for benefits
Consider quality of life, ethical issues and patient values
Use an active problem-solving approach involving the multi-professional team
Use evidence-based guidelines for managing symptoms

Agree on the simplest, most effective treatment regimen for that individual at that time

Constantly re-evaluate through continued dialogue with patient/family

with cancer is symptoms that arise as a consequence of their advanced disease (Kaye 1996, Twycross 1997, Regnard & Tempest 1998). People with other advanced progressive diseases are also likely to have symptoms, but this is less well evidenced (NCHSPCS 1998).

> Life threatening, progressing disease is a creeping crisis that invades patients, partners, and carers alike. Although some will grow from the experience, it remains a distressing experience for all.
> (Regnard & Tempest 1998)

Patients with symptoms can be found in all settings – home, hospital and hospice – although the majority of people spend 90% of their final year of life being cared for at home (Cartwright 1991). Throughout this time they are encouraged to live life to the full. However, the patient may be admitted for assessment and stabilisation of symptoms (Penson & Fisher 1995). Most people express the wish to die at home but only 25% of people do. Hinton (1994) wondered if people might change their mind as death approached. The reason most often given for admission to a palliative care unit or hospital is difficulty in controlling symptoms (Townsend et al 1990). It could be argued that other important issues are considered in the admission process but are, perhaps, not documented. For example, lack of provision of appropriate care and support, inability of the carer to cope, fear of the unknown and the patient requesting not to die at home.

The basic principles of symptom management apply, regardless of the setting. An interesting consideration is whether the setting in which the patient is being cared for has an influence on the incidence or severity of symptoms. Lay beliefs, sometimes regarded as unscientific and based on folklore or individual experience, can have a profound effect on the patients and their families' perceptions (Blaxter 1990). A family caring for the patient at home may be more alert to changing symptoms as they offer continuity of care and vigilance. Alternatively, the family may ignore symptoms as they think this heralds a deterioration in the condition and illustrates the inevitability of death.

Prevalence of symptoms

Studies establishing the prevalence of symptoms in patients with cancer are limited to selected populations, usually those patients who use a hospice service or oncology clinics. Evidence to explore the prevalence of symptoms in those patients with progressive non-malignant disease is scant, as it is confined to patients referred to a palliative care service (Higginson 1997). The Regional Study of Care for the dying examined the experiences of people in the last year of life who died from heart disease, stroke and cancer. The information was from bereaved relatives (Addington-Hall 1993). This study substantiates work by Cartwright (1991) and Seale (1991) that illustrates the prevalence of symptoms in a random sample of national deaths in 1987 and has been used to calculate the number of patients with symptoms as viewed by bereaved carers.

Table 4.1 shows a comparison of the findings for malignant and non-malignant disease.

Other symptoms known to be prevalent in malignant disease include (Kaye 1994):

- weakness 95%
- sweats 60%
- oedema 60%
- dry sore mouth 50%
- anxiety 40%
- cough 30%
- drowsiness 10%
- itch 5%

Multiple symptoms

Many patients have multiple symptoms. This factor increases patient anxiety and distress for the patient and family (Higginson 1997), which makes a symptom worse and more difficult to assess (Redmond 1996). The challenge of managing the patient with multiple symptoms is summarised by Desbiens (1997):

> Until we unravel the myriad of possible interconnections between symptoms, our treatment should be directed at relieving each symptom that can increase the burden of suffering in seriously ill patients.

Table 4.1 Comparison of malignant and non-malignant disease. (From Cartwright 1991, Seale 1991, Addington-Hall 1993)

Symptom	Patients with cancer (% with symptom in last year of life)	Patients with progressive non-malignant disease (% with symptom in last year of life)
Pain	84	67
Trouble with breathing	47	49
Vomiting or nausea	51	27
Sleeplessness	51	36
Mental confusion	33	38
Depression	38	36
Loss of appetite	71	38
Constipation	47	32
Bed sores	28	14
Loss of bladder control	37	33
Loss of bowel control	25	22
Unpleasant smell	19	32

Management of symptoms other than pain

To discuss the management of all symptoms other than pain is not possible in this chapter. The reading list suggests suitable texts. The authors explore the management of common symptoms through Case study 4.1.

MANAGING THE SYMPTOMS
Specific haematological symptoms

The value of blood and platelet transfusions as a supportive mode of treatment in haematology and oncology units is well established. However, its usefulness in palliative care may be less well recognised. Weakness, shortness of breath, fatigue and a general feeling of being less well are experienced by a significant proportion of patients with advanced malignancy, which is reflected in their quality of life (Gleeson & Spencer 1995). The focus of care is the comfort of the patients, not an ideal full blood count. Therefore, the necessity of transfusion should be based upon the patient's perception of distressing symptoms. Rationalising the use of platelet transfusion is a less contentious issue than the use of blood transfusion, as its adminis-

tration is a prophylactic measure to prevent bleeding.

Mouth care

The relevance and importance of identifying and managing oral symptoms in advanced disease and the associated distress has been highlighted in a number of studies (Addington-Hall & McCarthy 1995, Field et al 1995). Yet despite this evidence there is still the need for much research to identify effective management, as much of the rationale for addressing oral complications is practice-based evidence (Krishnasamy 1995). Tables 4.2, 4.3 and 4.4 outline the major problems encountered when managing oral symptoms and the associated interventions to address them. This is information adapted from the Further Reading at the end of the chapter and the following references: Blom et al (1996), Davies (1997) and Twycross & Back (1998).

Nausea and vomiting

Nausea and vomiting are common symptoms in advanced disease for which there are many causes. Successful treatment relies upon a careful history of the symptoms, combined with recent research about the mechanisms of nausea and

CASE STUDY 4.1

MANAGEMENT OF COMMON SYMPTOMS

Jean was a 47-year-old woman who had a busy responsible working life as a Chief Superintendent of Police. She lived with Hazel, her life partner, who is a retired superintendent policewoman. They had a comfortable life together in their own home in a rural area supported by a strong network of friends. They were financially secure. Jean was diagnosed with Philadelphia positive acute myeloblastic leukaemia in April 1995.

Chemotherapy achieved complete remission in August of the same year.

Jean relapsed in April 1996 and was given further chemotherapy. Jean and her family were informed about her poor prognosis. At best, remission could be achieved: Jean achieved remission.

In December 1996 she suffered a profound relapse. She was given chemotherapy and high-dose steroids but no significant improvement in the disease was evident.

Numerous admissions followed because of various infections. A wide range of antibiotics were given. As well as increased susceptibility to infection, Jean also had problems with persistent purpuric rash, and bleeding gums and teeth.

From April 1997 Jean was pancytopaenic, her marrow unrecoverable. She was requiring platelet transfusions at least three times each week and a blood transfusion every 7–10 days.

Physical symptoms at this time were:

- tiredness
- breathlessness
- fatigue
- purpuric rash
- mouth bleeding.

Most of these symptoms were addressed when she was given her regular blood products (packed cells and platelets).

At this point in time, Jean and Hazel explored their fears and anxieties surrounding Jean's death and about the possibility of being hospitalised unnecessarily with the Macmillan nurse. This was very important for both of them. At this time the assessment of her physical symptoms was coloured by her anxiety about admission to the hospital and the speed of her impending death. There was no

reason for her to be hospitalised at this time as they were managing very well at home.

Towards the end of June, which turned out to be the terminal phase of Jean's disease, she had a gastrointestinal bleed. An endoscopy confirmed a purpuric rash in the gastrointestinal tract. She also developed the following physical symptoms:

- worsening hepatosplenomegaly
- gastric stasis
- inferior vena caval obstruction resulting in severe oedema
- constipation
- sore mouth
- breathlessness
- weakness and fatigue.

Jean felt that this was the first time her physical frailty had affected the way she lived her life. Jean and Hazel were very tearful. They were most definite that they wished Jean's symptoms to be treated aggressively. Jean felt it was unacceptable to have such limited mobility as she had set tasks as goals, which required an increase in physical capabilities. They reiterated their wish to be cared for at home, yet accepted minimal input from the community services. A close friend was with them when extra support was needed.

There was an impression that Jean was deteriorating, although she was symptomatically much better. She said she felt better than she had for weeks. She achieved a good quality of life for 3 weeks, feeling relatively well and travelling daily to the hospital for platelet support.

She became very weak, with what appeared to be a proximal myopathy due to the prolonged use of steroids. Within the last few days of her life she was unable to travel for platelet support to the hospital and was nursed at home by Hazel and her friends, with help from community services.

Hazel discussed the conditional change with the approach of death and was able to rationalise Jean's medication, stopping some and changing others to a non-oral route. Jean remained awake until the last 12 hours of her life. Hazel and her friends nursed her beautifully in her final days, with the nurse specialists and district nurse visiting her at home to help as needed.

Jean showed how palliative care can improve quality of life and assist the patient to a peaceful death in the place of their choice.

---

vomiting being applied to clinical practice (Regnard & Hockley 1995). It is now accepted that there are three main pathways that trigger nausea and vomiting (Mannix 1997, Twycross 1997, Twycross & Back 1998):

1. chemoreceptor trigger zone – CTZ – chemical triggers
2. vomiting centre – VC – cerebral trigger and/or visceral trigger
3. gastrointestinal disturbances.

Table 4.2   Care of dry mouth

Subject	Likely cause	Intervention
Dry mouth	Caused by the cancer, e.g. direct invasion Local radiotherapy Local radical surgery Chemotherapy Drug therapy, e.g. opioids, anticholinergics Oxygen therapy Dehydration Anxiety Mouth breathing Infection, e.g. candidiasis Concurrent disorders, e.g. diabetes mellitus Combination of above	Encourage regular sips of water Review current drug regimen Stimulate salivary flow using: • chewing gum • ice chips • citrus fruit drinks • acid/lemon sweets • 2% citric acid solution • ascorbic acid tablets • acupuncture Pilocarpine – stimulates secretion of saliva, protects oral mucosa and increases mucin in saliva Use of artificial salivary agents Gin and tonic, ice cubes

Table 4.3   Care of painful mouth

Subject	Likely cause	Intervention
Painful mouth	Cytotoxic drugs Radiotherapy	Topical analgesics • 5% lignocaine paste • benzydamine mouthwash or spray (may cause stinging) • choline salicylate gel • dispersible aspirin mouthwash Sucralfate suspension as a protective agent
	Candidiasis	Clean mouth well Nystatin suspension or pastilles Miconazole gel Ketoconazole or fluconazole Amphotericin lozenges Prophylactic therapy in the immunocompromised patient Treat dentures overnight
	Aphthous ulceration	Chlorhexidine gluconate 0.2% mouthwash Tetracycline suspension Choline salicylate gel Carbenoxolone Triamcinolone paste Benzocaine lozenges 2.5% hydrocortisone pellets Thalidomide for severe aphthous ulceration

Administering drugs by the non-oral route

If vomiting is preventing drug absorption via the oral route, or if the patient is persistently nauseated, the use of alternative modes of delivery is necessary. These may include the rectal or subcutaneous route. If the drug is administered subcutaneously, continuous subcutaneous infusion preceded by an immediate dose or regular injection via an indwelling subcutaneous cannula is preferable. The drug may be given by mouth once the symptom is under control.

The psychological approach

Persistent nausea and vomiting is a very debilitating problem. The anxiety caused by associated weight loss and weakness can increase the fear the patient may experience. A psychological approach to reduce this windup mechanism may be beneficial. Table 4.5 outlines the management of nausea and vomiting.

Weakness and fatigue

Fatigue is a common symptom in advanced disease. Some studies illustrate that it is one of the

Table 4.4   Care of dirty mouth

Subject	Likely cause	Intervention
Dirty mouth	Poor oral hygiene	Regular teeth brushing Rinse mouth well Use electric toothbrush if dexterity is poor Chlorhexidine mouthwash Suck or chew pineapple chunks Dissolve effervescent vitamin C on the tongue Cider and soda water mouthwash Sodium perborate (Bocasan) mouthwash Soft toothbrush and: • hydrogen peroxide • sodium bicarbonate • sodium chloride 0.9%
	Gastritis	Treat mouth as above and gastritis with antacids or H$_2$ antagonists

Table 4.5   Management of nausea and vomiting

Symptom	Likely cause	Intervention
Nausea and vomiting	Chemoreceptor trigger zone (CTZ): • metabolic disturbance • drugs • sepsis • alcohol	Haloperidol Ondansetron for chemotherapy-induced vomiting Treat any reversible causes
	Vomiting centre (VC) • Cerebral triggers: anxiety fear pain external stimuli, e.g. smells anticipatory vomiting • Visceral triggers: stretched organs distorted organs, e.g. raised intracranial pressure, motion sickness, constipation and ascites	Cyclizine Hyoscine hydrobromide Ondansetron Acupressure wrist bands Acupuncture Psychological support +/- sedatives Prokinetic agents, including: • metoclopramide (upper gut) • domperidone (upper gut) • cisapride (upper and lower gut) Antacids H$_2$ antagonists
	Gastrointestinal disturbance: • constipation • gastric stasis • partial bowel obstruction • radiotherapy to the gut • gastritis • peptic ulceration • food poisoning	

most disturbing symptoms reported by patients, as it causes the greatest amount of interference with self-care (Rhodes et al 1988). Fatigue is multifactorial and multidimensional: the biological, psychological, social and personal factors all affect the patient's experience (Richardson 1995). Table 4.6 outlines interventions which may be employed to address this symptom.

Inferior vena caval obstruction

Advanced disease may result in compression or occlusion of venous blood flow, with a resultant accumulation of fluid in the genitals, lower limbs and tissues of the lower trunk. There are several reasons for this; however, in Jean's case (Case study 4.1), hepatosplenomegaly as a result of advanced haematological disease was the main causative factor (Mortimer et al 1995).

This may be managed as follows:

1. High-dose steroids. These may reduce visceral swelling, in turn reducing the degree of obstruction, which results in reduced oedema.
2. Diuretic therapy. Commencement of diuretics or manipulation of an existing regimen may aid the excretion of fluid and alleviate oedema.
3. Measurement of the serum albumin. Hypoalbumenaemia (low protein) may exacerbate oedema. The administration of albumin with high-dose diuretics may be effective.

Table 4.7 Laxatives. (Adapted from Fallon & O'Neill 1997, Sykes 1997, Twycross 1997, Maestri-Banks 1998)

Category	Type of laxative	Laxative and description
Predominantly faecal-softening laxatives	Surfactants	Increase water penetration and soften the stool
		Take 1–3 days to work
		Co-danthramer-poloxamer and danthron
		Co-danthrusate-danthron and docusate
		Both of the above are a combination of softener and stimulant and are effective for opioid-induced constipation
	Osmotics	Flush small bowel; large doses may cause colic and bloating
		Require an increase in fluid intake
		Lactulose is frequently used but causes flatulence and is very sweet
		Sorbitol is less sweet
	Bulk-forming	Really are stool normalisers
		Require great increase in fluid intake
		Fybogel increases faecal mass
	Saline	Bran can enhance dietary intake
	lubricants	Magnesium sulphate for rapid evacuation
		May fail to produce rectal stimulation
		Liquid paraffin – rarely used; causes irritation
Predominantly peristalsis-stimulating laxatives		Stimulate the mesenteric plexus to induce peristalsis
		Good for opioid-induced constipation
		Can cause colic
		Senna and danthron both effective given with a softener
		Danthron can turn the urine pink or red; observe for a perianal rash
Combination laxatives		As above, combination products include:
		Co-danthramer
		Co-danthramer strong
		Co-danthrusate
		Millpar

disordered breathing. Dyspnoea is more common and often more severe in the last few weeks of life. Patients who are dyspnoeic are more likely to be anxious (Twycross 1997).

Assessment

Breathlessness is common in advanced disease. Careful individualised, multi-professional assessment is essential. Assessment involves a detailed history of the pattern of breathlessness, predisposing factors and associated feelings of panic, fear and anxiety. Corner et al (1996) identify a paucity of research into dyspnoea in advanced cancer. There has been a failure to address dyspnoea as a complex symptom with a wide variety of causes. Therapeutic interventions are often focussed on a pharmacological approach. Corner et al (1996)

advocate an integrative model of dyspnoea, illustrating the need to move beyond current models of intervention. Their model leads to an holistic understanding of breathlessness (Fig. 4.1).

Causes of dyspnoea in advanced cancer

Causes of dyspnoea in advanced cancer are given in Table 4.8 which is adapted from Twycross (1997).

Treat the underlying cause

It is essential that all medical and surgical interventions have been undertaken. For example, if there is established chronic obstructive pulmonary disease (COPD) a bronchodilator may help. Ensure that all antitumour therapy has

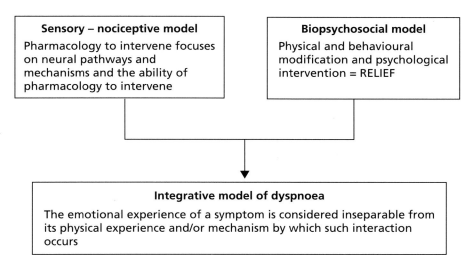

Figure 4.1   Integrative model of dyspnoea.

been given; chemotherapy, radiotherapy, laser treatment or stenting may be of assistance. All treatment options must be explored and a multi-disciplinary approach adopted.

Management options

The pharmacological and non-pharmacological strategies commonly adopted are illustrated in Table 4.9.

The effects on dyspnoea on quality of life can be immense. It directly affects the person's ability to perform all activities and can promote intense anxiety (Corner et al 1995).

MANAGING SYMPTOMS IN THE TERMINAL PHASE

When is the terminal phase?

Recognising the last days or hours of a patient's life is not always easy, even for experienced professionals. A recent study showed that a nursing auxiliary was able to more accurately predict imminent death than other health professionals (Oxenham & Cornbleet 1998). Physical and behavioural changes that occur over weeks or days may provide clues. For most patients, a gradual weakening occurs as the body's vital functions fail to cope and the patient becomes

Table 4.8   Causes of dyspnoea in advanced cancer. (Adapted from Twycross 1997)

Caused by cancer	Caused by treatment	Related to cancer	Concurrent causes and/or debility
Pleural effusion(s)	Radiation-induced fibrosis	Anaemia	COPD (chronic obstructive pulmonary disease)
Obstruction of the main bronchus	Chemotherapy, e.g. bleomycin	Atelectasis	Asthma
Cancer in lung		Pulmonary embolism	Heart failure
Lymphangitis carcinomatosis		Pneumonia	Acidosis
Mediastinal obstruction		Empyema	
Pericardial effusion		Cachexia-anorexia syndrome	
Massive ascites		Weakness	
Abdominal distension			

Table 4.9 Strategies used to treat dyspnoea. (Adapted from Kaye 1997, Twycross 1997, Booth 1999)

Symptom	Pharmacological management	Non-pharmacological management
Breath-lessness	Morphine – opioids reduce ventilatory responses to hypoxia and hypercapnia Steroids – useful in lymphangitis and metastatic disease Oxygen Benzodiazepines – diazepam, lorazepam and midazolam Nebulised opiates – scant evidence to suggest these are any better than saline Cannabinoids, e.g. nabilone, good for patients in respiratory failure	A palliative approach Calm and confident manner Reassurance Cool stream of air Physiotherapy Breathing exercises Address fear and anxiety Relaxation Complementary therapy Massage Hypnosis Acupuncture Cognitive behavioural therapy Education Adaptation of the activities of daily living

unconscious, leading to respiratory and cardiac failure and death. These changes may include some or all of the following:

- *Altered appearance* – translucency and faded colour of skin; cool cyanosed extremities; lank hair; greasy sweat; gaunt facial features; cartilage of ears and nose are pale and prominent; eyes become glazed, distant and hollow.
- *Decreased physical functioning* – profound weakness; whispering voice; increased dependency; increased tiredness and longer periods of sleep; disinterest in food and fluids; continence problems.
- *Change in mental functioning* – poor concentration; preoccupation or vagueness; reduced response to outside stimuli; disorientation; confusion; restlessness.
- *Altered vital signs* – changes in pulse and breathing rate, rhythm and volume.
- *Other changes* – loss of interest or engagement in social interaction; focus on memories of those who have already died; insignificance of

difference between night and day; voices knowledge of impending death; makes farewells with loved ones.

Sudden deterioration over a few days should prompt a search for potentially reversible causes: for example, hypercalcaemia, infection or side effects from changes in medication.

Why is symptom management different at this stage?

Having identified that the terminal phase has begun, the principles of symptom management should be the same as at any other stage of the patient's illness. The patient may no longer be capable of participating in treatment and care decisions. The family may be more anxious and distressed by the symptoms than previously (Holing 1986). Family observations of the patient's experience may also now be influenced by their own fears about death (NCHSPCS 1997). The patient *may* not be able to be involved in decisions. The aims and outcomes of treatments are altered as death approaches.

Ethical and legal issues come sharply into focus, as the patient's weakened state prompts discussions about the benefits of continuing treatments and attempting to maintain comfort without shortening or ending life. Pressure on health professionals is increased by the growing number of medical litigation cases and the number of times that the guidance of the court has been sought on the treatment of vulnerable patients. Voluntary euthanasia and advance directives have also been prominent in the media in recent years. Consequently, staff fears and anxieties can influence the decisions made about care in the terminal phase (NCHSPCS 1997). These ethical and legal issues are discussed in more detail in Chapter 14 but it is important to remember that:

Ultimately the real protection of the vulnerable ill lies not so much in a highly vigilant legal system (which cannot possibly police every case) but in the ethical sense of those who provide medical care.

(Byrne 1993)

Anxiety and distress in both the family and professionals can cloud their ability to assess and plan appropriate care unless it is recognised that death approaches. This phase requires redefinition of goals and reappraisal of treatments and symptom control, a 'gear change' (NCHSPCS 1997). It is important to communicate and explain the patient's changing condition to the family so that they may understand changing approaches to care. This is prompted by several factors, including the patient's increasing difficulty taking oral medication; inability to cooperate with care; disinterest in activity; and increased need for rest and sleep.

Reassessment of symptoms is important at this stage as patients' tolerance of previous symptoms may be poor due to their debility and they may develop new symptoms (Conill et al 1997; NCHSPCS 1997).

The main aims of care, now, are maintenance of comfort and dignity, palliation of distressing symptoms and improvement of the quality of the remaining time. The appropriateness of treatment and care need to be reviewed with this in mind. Byrne (1993) suggests that it can be useful to consider the difference between productive treatment, that is treatment which does not exacerbate or prolong suffering and provides real hope for the future, and non-productive treatment. It is generally inappropriate to offer futile treatment even if it is requested. The patient who has been taking long-term medication for angina or hypertension is unlikely to benefit from this medication in the terminal phase and the treatment could be stopped. Similarly, hormone treatment for breast cancer is of no benefit at this stage. Other treatments that do need to be continued, such as analgesics or antiemetics, may need to be given by a different route if the patient cannot swallow. If tolerance of existing symptoms is poor, current treatments may need to be changed. These changes need careful explanation, so that the family understands the reason. Misunderstandings about motives for changing therapy may lead to them feeling that professionals have given up or are attempting to hasten death.

Management of specific symptoms that occur in the last days or hours

Symptoms such as nausea, vomiting or dyspnoea will probably persist in this stage and

Table 4.10 Management of terminal restlessness, agitation and confusion

Symptom	Likely cause	Management
Restlessness/agitation (without confusion)	Mostly myoclonic jerks from: • Uraemia • liver failure • drugs, e.g. opiates • drug withdrawal • cerebral, e.g. metastases/hypoxia	Benzodiazepine by non-oral route, e.g. midazolam subcutaneously Anticonvulsants, e.g. barbiturates Explanation to relatives that this is not necessarily a sign of distress
(a) Involuntary spontaneous movement		
(b) Coordinated movements: 'tossing and turning' or 'fumbling'	Physical discomfort – pain, full bladder, constipation, nausea, dyspnoea	Treat cause, try simple remedies first; e.g. offer bedpan, sit upright to maximise chest expansion
(c) Confusion with or without restlessness (mental disturbances – poor comprehension, hallucinations, misperceptions, disorientation, etc.)	Metabolic – organ failure • hypercalcaemia • hyponatraemia • hypoglycaemia Hypoxia Infection Cerebral metastases Drugs Constipation Previous psychiatric diagnosis	Treatment of causes may be appropriate even at this late stage purely for comfort; e.g. antibiotics can reduce fever and toxicity A quiet calm environment and continued explanation to patient and family Soothing physical therapy; e.g. massage and aromatherapy Sedation with benzodiazepine or phenothiazine

may be worse. Medication should be continued and converted to a non-oral route if necessary. The most commonly reported symptoms, other than pain, which occur at the end of life are dyspnoea, nausea and vomiting, confusion, agitation, restlessness, noisy breathing, urinary incontinence, retention of urine, dry and sore mouth and extreme fatigue (Fainsinger et al 1991, Conill et al 1997, NCHSPCS 1997). This section will specifically address the management of agitation and restlessness, confusion, noisy breathing and dry mouth in the terminal phase.

Agitation, restlessness and confusion

In the final days or hours, some patients will seem unable to settle, with constant limb movements. This can be distressing for the patient and family and staff. It is important to distinguish between restlessness, agitation and confusion, as management differs. Physical restraint is not helpful, as it increases feelings of unfamiliarity. Restriction may cause falls if the patient tries to break free (Twycross 1997). As with other symptoms, explanation of possible causes and intended treatment will help to allay anxiety and distress. Table 4.10 shows how to distinguish between these symptoms and some interventions that will help.

Noisy breathing

This is often referred to as death rattle and is reported to occur in 56–92% of dying patients (Bennett 1996, Watts et al 1997). It is caused by a build-up of secretions in the pharynx or trachea that vibrate or bubble with respiration. The secretions may come from salivary glands when the swallowing reflex is poor or from bronchial mucosa when the cough reflex is lost. Excessive bronchial secretions arise if the patient has a respiratory infection or heart failure.

Although this is a common problem in the terminal phase and is reported to be distressing for families and staff, it is difficult to know how much it distresses patients. Family distress may be compounded by their need to see the patient comfort-able. Noisy breathing may suggest discomfort. This symptom has not been well researched and much of the literature is anecdotal (Watts et al 1997). Staff distress may be increased by poor confidence in managing this symptom due to the absence of evidence-based effective interventions.

Management includes:

- explanation to relatives
- positioning the patient to encourage postural drainage of secretions
- gentle suction, using a soft catheter
- anticholinergic drugs: for example, hyoscine hydrobromide or glycopyrronium, if salivary secretions are the cause
- diuretics, which may help if the cause is thought to be pulmonary oedema.

Anticholinergic drugs are more successful when used for salivary secretions than bronchial secretions and need to be administered at the first sign of excess secretions as they only prevent further secretion. They do not remove secretions which are already present.

Mouthcare

Despite dry mouth being frequently cited as a common and distressing symptom in the terminal phase, research into effective care is rare and current interventions are based on practice-based evidence (Jenkins 1997, Krishnasamy 1995).

Family or carers may think that the patient is dehydrated or 'dying of thirst'. There is much debate among health professionals and the general public about the need for parenteral fluids at the end of life and there is some evidence that there are differences in the approach to this according to the setting. House (1992) found that hospital staff were more likely to allow their own fears about ethical and legal issues to guide the treatment decision than hospice staff. This is an ongoing emotive debate in which the principles of productive and non-productive treatments can be used to establish the likely benefits for each individual. It can be helpful to assess the patient for other signs and symptoms of dehydration – for example, confusion, dizziness and dry skin. According to Ellershaw et al (1995), there is no significant association between the level of hydration and symptoms of thirst and dry mouth. Only if other symptoms of dehydration are present and the patient is distressed, should parenteral fluid administration be considered. The potential relief of dizziness and confusion needs to be balanced with the possible distress which may result from increased secretions, a need to pass urine more frequently and the use of invasive equipment. It can be hard to remember that the patient is dying and the aim is to relieve discomfort, not to ensure that the patient has a perfect fluid balance chart or electrolyte balance (Twycross 1997).

If parenteral fluid is required, a subcutaneous or intravenous infusion could be administered. The subcutaneous route is useful if an intravenous infusion would be difficult. Subcutaneous injection of hyaluronidase before the infusion and once every 24 hours will promote absorption of fluid from subcutaneous tissues (Noble-Adams 1995).

The patient may not be able to swallow well and cooperation with mouthwashes and brushing teeth will be difficult, so many interventions mentioned in the section 'Managing the symptoms' will not be possible. The aim of care is to moisten the patient's mouth and prevent damage to the oral mucosa or lips. If the patient is unconscious, care will be needed at least hourly (Krishnasamy 1995), and can be carried out by the family if they wish to be involved, although some may find this distressing.

Useful interventions include:

- Clean the patient's mouth using chlorhexidine solution on sponge sticks or a gauze-wrapped finger. A solution of equal parts of cider and soda water is also effective, and has a pleasant taste. Hydrogen peroxide has been shown to have an unpleasant taste and can cause stinging and nausea (Krishnasamy 1995).
- Moisten the mouth with water-soaked cloth, gauze or a sponge stick or place small ice chips on the tongue. Alternatives to water are tonic water, with or without gin, and citrus-based fruit juices, as both of these can stimulate saliva. Glycerine-based products are not useful, as they dry the oral mucosa (Krishnasamy 1995).

- Moisturise the patient's lips with Vaseline or moisturising lotion to prevent chapping.

Syringe drivers

Subcutaneous infusions are a useful way of administering medication once the patient is unable to manage oral medication and avoids the use of multiple injections. There are many models of syringe driver and each has a unique set of instructions. Most care institutions will also have their own guidelines for choosing sites, dressings and observations: for example, the *Royal Marsden Manual of Clinical Nursing Procedures* (Pritchard & Mallet 1994).

Practical tips:

- The compatibility of diamorphine with antiemetics or sedatives has been investigated and few instances of instability have been found when infusions are changed every 24 hours (Allwood 1984, Allwood et al 1994, Twycross 1997). There seems to be no consensus on the number of agents which can be mixed in a syringe and maintain stability. Some specialists in palliative care have made recommendations for no more than two drugs to be mixed (Regnard & Tempest 1998) while others recommend no more than three (Ellershaw 1996). *Advice should be sought from a pharmacist.*
- Crystallisation can occur with cyclizine in combination with certain salts – for example, chloride and bromide. It should be mixed with water for injections and observed closely, particularly if mixed with diamorphine, hyoscine hydrobromide or metoclopramide.
- The injection site may become inflamed more quickly than usual when infusing levomepromazine or cyclizine. Observation should be frequent. Hydrocortisone cream (1%) can alleviate irritation.

CONCLUSION

Nurses are important members of the multidisciplinary team and play a major role in promoting comfort for the patient with symptoms other than pain. Identifying patients' problems and using research-based strategies to prevent, allevi-

doctors' attitudes towards patients' wishes and euthanasia. Medical Journal of Australia 165: 540–544

Watts T, jenkins K, Back I 1997 Problem and mangement of noisy rattling breathing in dying patients. International Journal of Palliative Nursing 3: 245–252

Wilkinson 1991 Factors which influence how nurses communicate with cancer patients. Journal of Advanced Nursing 16: 177–188

Wilson-Barnett J, Batehup L 1988 Patient problems: a research base for nursing care. Scutari Press, London

FURTHER READING

Back I 1997 Palliative medicine handbook. Holme Tower Marie Curie Centre, Penarth, Wales

Doyle D, Hanks G, Macdonald G 1995 Oxford textbook of palliative medicine, 2nd edn. Oxford University Press, Oxford

Kaye P 1996 A–Z pocketbook of symptoms. EPL Publications, Northampton

Kaye P 1997 Tutorials in palliative medicine. EPL Publications, Northampton

National Council for Hospice and Specialist Palliative Care Services (NCHSPCS). Various publications available from their offices in UK

Penson J, Fisher R 1995 Palliative care for people with cancer, 2nd edn. Arnold, London

Regnard C, Hockley J 1995 Flow diagrams in advanced cancer and other diseases. Edward Arnold, London

Regnard C, Tempest S 1998 A guide to symptom relief in advanced disease, 4th edn. Hochland and Hochland, Cheshire

Twycross R 1997 Symptom management in advanced cancer, 2nd edn. Radcliffe Medical Press, Oxford

5

Promoting comfort through surgery, chemotherapy and radiotherapy

Philippa Green   James Youll

INTRODUCTION

In this chapter we examine how to support patients while they are receiving palliative care. We discuss the management and possible side effects experienced by patients undergoing palliative radiotherapy and chemotherapy. We outline the indications for the use of palliative surgery and explore radiological interventions including use of stents. A case study illustrates the value of the above techniques where traditional palliative surgery may be difficult or impossible. It is often difficult to imagine radiotherapy or chemotherapy being used in palliative care, especially if we have experience of caring for patients who have undergone treatment with curative intent. These patients may experience side effects which are often severe but tolerated because of the overall aim of treatment. When we examine the palliative use of chemotherapy and radiotherapy, thorough assessment must take place before and throughout treatment. Nurses are often in the best position to identify symptoms and aid diagnosis as well as assess the overall effects of treatment, in conjunction with the patient and family.

Hoskin (1994) states: 'Palliative treatment is delivered with the intent of achieving control of local symptoms in a setting where cure is no longer possible, using treatment designed to give minimal disturbance to the lifestyle of the patient.'

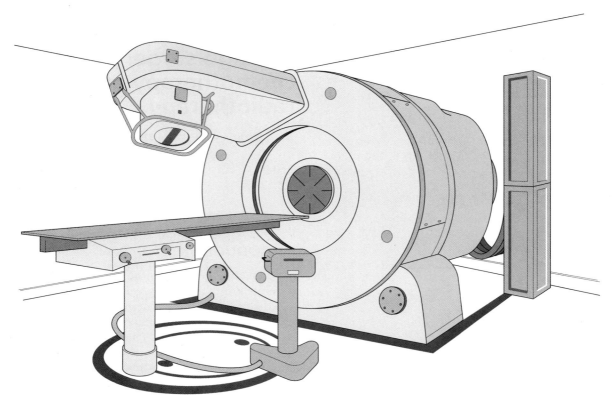

Figure 5.1   Diagram of linear accelerator, reprinted from Cancer and Radiotherapy, 2nd edn, Walter, J., Linear accelerator for megavoltage therapy, p. 60, 1977, with kind permission of Churchill Livingstone.

WHAT IS RADIOTHERAPY?

Radiotherapy is the use of ionising radiation to interfere with the replication of cancer cells within the body. Radiotherapy cannot differentiate between normal cells and cancer cells, so normal cells will be affected within the path of the radiation beam, causing the patient to experience side effects (Green & Kinghorn 1995, Kirkbride 1995, Holmes 1996a, Robinson & Coleman 1996).

Most radiotherapy departments use machines called linear accelerators, which generate radiation using electricity (Fig. 5.1). However, there are still some departments with machines that utilise radioactive material, usually cobalt. Kirkbride (1995) points out that, despite the different applications, the effects of the treatment will be the same.

Radiotherapy can be given using these machines, or by placing radioactive material into the tissue or into a cavity close to the site of the cancer. This treatment is known as brachytherapy. Radioactive isotopes can be administered either by mouth or intravenous injection to carry out investigations or to treat certain cancers. All of these techniques can be used to treat cancer curatively or palliatively.

Palliative radiotherapy

The decision to treat curatively or palliatively is well thought out by the consultant clinical oncologist, taking into account the extent of the disease, the physical and personal circumstances of patients and their wishes.

Sometimes, at diagnosis, it may be evident that the disease is so extensive that cure may be impossible. It may seem strange to be considering radiotherapy as a palliative treatment because of side effects but it has been shown to be useful in managing patients who experience distressing symptoms and for whom cure is no longer possible. It has been estimated that approximately 45% of patients with cancer will receive radiotherapy at some time during their illness (Robinson & Coleman 1996) and that approximately half of radiotherapy treatments are given with palliative intent (Kirkbride 1995).

The overall doses of radiotherapy used for palliative treatments are lower than those given with curative intent and the delivery can range from a single exposure to several fractions spread over a period of up to 2 weeks. While giving palliative treatment the aim is to maintain or enhance quality of life.

Continuous monitoring of the effects of the treatment on the patient and their carers is important. Nursing staff within hospital, community and nursing homes are relied upon to report any adverse effects to medical staff directly involved with the patient or to the radiographers within the department who can relay information to the appropriate staff.

Symptoms that may be alleviated by radiotherapy, side effects and their management

Brain metastases

Breast cancer, small-cell lung cancer, melanoma and renal cancer commonly metastasise to the brain as well as AIDS-related cerebral lymphoma. In these cases palliative radiotherapy produces a reasonable response (Neal & Hoskin 1997). Presenting symptoms of brain metastases may include headache, blurred vision, ataxia and possible seizures (Waller & Caroline 1996).

Patients initially start high doses of corticosteroids to reduce intracranial pressure and relieve cerebral oedema (Souhami & Tobias 1998). Radiotherapy is a useful mode of treatment in patients with brain metastases and the response to treatment relates to the radiosensitivity of the primary cancer and to the response to corticosteroids.

Radiotherapy can be given to the whole brain if multiple deposits are present or treatment can be directed towards a single deposit.

Chemotherapy may also produce a response in metastases where the primary cancer is chemosensitive. Ongoing studies to identify a drug which may 'open' the blood–brain barrier to be given in conjunction with cytotoxic chemotherapy offer hope, although these studies have not been fully evaluated at present.

Bone metastases

The development of bone metastases is common in cancers such as breast, prostate, thyroid and lung (O'Brien 1993). Waller & Caroline (1996) state that there is a 30–70% incidence of bone metastases in all patients with cancer.

Assessment and prompt identification are important as the patient can experience severe bone pain and, untreated, there is an increased risk of pathological fracture. Presenting signs of bone metastases are pain, hypercalcaemia and pathological fracture; 85% of patients with bony metastases will suffer pain (Richardson 1989), which is made worse by hypercalcaemia.

Bone metastases and associated pain are generally very responsive to radiotherapy (O'Brien 1993), with some patients reporting an improvement within days. However, the duration of response varies. Radiotherapy can be given as a single exposure. The dose is fairly high and any side effects may be intense for a short period of time. The radiotherapy may be given over 5–10 days. If the treatment is to a long bone, such as the humerus or femur, the problems are limited, whereas treatment to the ribs or pelvis may be associated with more side effects because of underlying sensitive structures.

If the metastases are present in a long bone there is increased risk of pathological fracture. An orthopaedic consultation may be sought with a view to internal fixation. The patient will benefit from additional pain relief as a result of the internal fixation and mobility will be maintained or regained. Radiotherapy can be given follow-ing pinning (Smith 1993). Some patients may present with widespread bone metastases: if this occurs, they can be treated with hemi-body radi-ation, as a single exposure (Copp 1991). Again, the effects will depend upon which half of the body has been treated. A premedication of an antiemetic and a corticosteroid is usually given. Once a patient has completed a course of radio-therapy to manage pain, the patient's analgesic regimen will be reviewed.

Radioisotopes can also be used to treat bone metastases. Strontium-89 is a beta-emitting iso-tope which works by following the biochemical pathways of calcium. Given by injection it targets bony deposits and delivers radiotherapy locally, causing little damage to surrounding normal tis-sue (Needham 1997, Day 1998).

Until recently strontium was only licensed to treat bone pain in men with cancer of the prostate (Kaye 1994), but breast cancer patients may also benefit (Day 1998). Because the radioactive iso-tope is given intravenously the strontium is excreted via the kidneys so the patient's urine will be radioactive for a period of time. Patients who are incontinent of urine will require special medical consideration.

With both hemi-body irradiation and stron-tium, bone marrow suppression can be a prob-lem. Patient and family education is important with particular reference to control of infection.

Oral or intravenous bisphosphonates may be prescribed in the management of malignant hypercalcaemia (Fleisch 1995). They work by inhibiting bone resorption (Needham 1997, Souhami & Tobias 1998). Pamidronate can be used to treat hypercalcaemia in breast cancer patients and is given intravenously on a 4-weekly basis. It can also help in the management of bone metastases, reducing pain, fractures and the need for analgesia, while enhancing quality of life (O'Brien 1993).

Spinal cord compression (SCC)

Metastatic spread from breast cancer, cancer of the bronchus, lymphoma, prostate cancer, melanoma and unknown primary to the spinal cord is common (Waller & Caroline 1996, Souhami & Tobias 1998). It can be caused by bone metastases eroding the vertebral prominences or the cord itself may be involved. Presenting symptoms include altered sensation, pain and muscular weakness. Loss of sphincter control is a late symptom. SCC may be treated with surgical decompression followed by radiotherapy (Souhami & Tobias 1998).

As with other metastatic disease, response to radiotherapy may be determined by the radiosensitivity of the primary tumour. It is also dependent on the progression of the cord com-pression at the time of diagnosis. The earlier treatment can be initiated, the better the chance of patients retaining their mobility. The side effects caused by the radiotherapy will depend

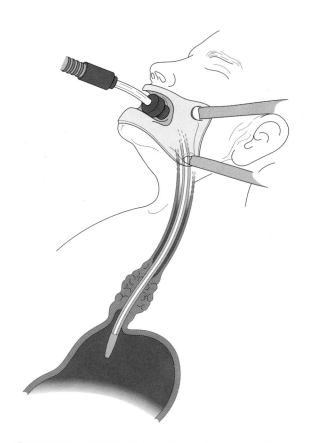

Figure 5.2a Treatment of oesophageal cancer using intraluminal brachytherapy, with kind permission of Nucletron.

on the area being treated. Chemotherapy may be of benefit but only if the primary tumour is known to be responsive to chemotherapy.

Spinal cord compression is considered as an oncological emergency. Rapid diagnosis, assessment and treatment are essential if neurological damage is not to become permanent (Coleman 1996a).

Oesophageal stricture

This is caused by a cancerous growth obstructing the oesophagus and can be treated palliatively in a number of ways. Surgical bypass may be an option, or the placement of a tube or a stent to allow the patient to maintain some oral intake of fluids (Souhami & Tobias 1998). Stenting is covered in more depth later in the chapter. Laser therapy can be used in conjunction with radiotherapy, although long-term evaluation is still awaited (Souhami & Tobias 1998).

Modest doses of radiotherapy can produce worthwhile results. The radiotherapy can be given externally over 1–2 weeks or it can be given as brachytherapy; this involves passing a tube into the oesophagus and introducing a high-activity radioactive source (Kirkbride 1995) using remote after-loading techniques (Fig. 5.2a). Radiotherapy centres may use different insertion techniques, but this procedure may be carried out on an outpatient basis depending on the patient's condition. Some patients may experience oesophagitis – the management is discussed later in this chapter.

Lung cancer

The nature and extent of the disease at diagnosis means that much of the care given is palliative. This can involve radiotherapy, chemotherapy or laser therapy. Only a small proportion of patients are cured and surgery offers the best chance of this.

Haemoptysis, cough and chest pain respond well to radiotherapy (Neal & Hoskin 1997, Needham 1997, Souhami & Tobias 1998).

Radiotherapy can be given as a short course of external treatment, ranging from 1 to 4 weeks or

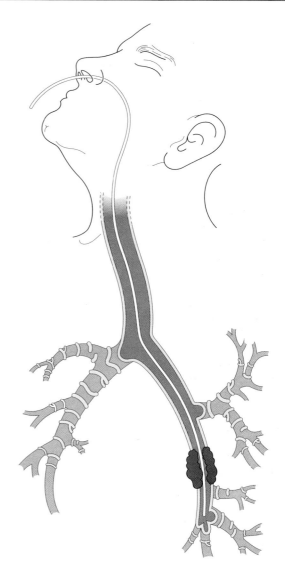

Figure 5.2b Treatment of bronchial cancer using intraluminal brachytherapy, with kind permission of Nucletron.

by using intraluminal brachytherapy (Needham 1997). A similar procedure to oesophageal brachytherapy is used. The patient will have tubes inserted into the bronchioles using a bronchoscope. A highly radioactive source is introduced into the tubes (Fig. 5.2b).

Laser therapy is useful to manage haemoptysis. It can be used when the patient has received the maximum tolerated dose of radiotherapy to the thorax (Heyse-Moore 1993, Neal & Hoskin 1997, Souhami & Tobias 1998). Silicone or expandable metal stents can be used to relieve tracheobronchial obstruction and dyspnoea (Heyse-Moore 1993).

Superior vena cava obstruction

Another oncological emergency is superior vena cava obstruction (SVCO), which results from pressure on the vessels from a tumour in the chest or mediastinum or secondary to thrombosis.

Carcinoma of the bronchus is the commonest primary cancer causing SVCO but breast cancer and lymphomas are also implicated (Coleman 1996a). The presenting signs are swelling of the face, neck and arms, engorgement of the jugular vein and dilatation of superficial skin veins, breathlessness, headaches and blurred vision (Coleman 1996a, Neal & Hoskin 1997, Souhami & Tobias 1998).

Treatment usually consists of radiotherapy combined with high-dose corticosteroids that are aimed at preventing an inflammatory reaction to the radiotherapy which would exacerbate the symptoms. The high-dose corticosteroids will need to be reduced carefully and quickly to prevent complications. The radiotherapy may be given as a short course or possibly over 4 weeks, depending on the primary diagnosis (Souhami & Tobias 1998). Chemotherapy may be considered if the primary tumour is chemosensitive.

Radiological stenting of the superior vena cava vessels has become possible and offers a valuable alternative to radiotherapy. It is a useful option if the problem recurs (Neal & Hoskin 1997).

Fungating tumours

A fungating cancer is a primary or secondary malignant growth in the skin which has ulcerated and which results in pain, exudate, bleeding, infection and malodour (Twycross 1997). These are common in patients with breast, vulval or penile cancers and some head and neck cancers. The wound may have the appearance of a raised nodule or an ulcerated crater with a distinct margin (Moody & Grocott 1993). Because of the extent of the growth, treatment will only be palliative but surgery may be considered, depending upon the site involved.

Often a combined approach using a topical antibiotic agent such as metronidazole gel and radiotherapy is used. Metronidazole helps to reduce malodour and treats infection caused by anaerobic bacteria. Radiotherapy reduces tumour bulk and the amount of exudate produced.

Sucralfate gel can also be used in the management of both fungating tumours and surface bleeding (Regnard & Tempest 1992, Waller & Caroline 1996, Twycross 1997).

Hormone therapy may be used and can help if the primary cancer is sensitive to hormone manipulation.

Haemorrhage

Non-acute bleeding can occur with some cancers as the growth erodes through smaller blood vessels. This can be seen as haemoptysis, vaginal bleeding, haematuria and rectal bleeding (Kaye 1994). Hoy (1993) describes radiotherapy as the most useful oncological treatment for tumour-related haemorrhage.

Radiotherapy can be given externally or by using brachytherapy techniques. As previously discussed brachytherapy can be used to treat haemoptysis. Brachytherapy techniques can also be used to treat vaginal bleeding from gynaecological cancer. Whale (1991) says that radiotherapy has an important role in palliating symptoms such as vaginal bleeding and pain. An applicator is placed into the vagina and uterus, into which radioactive sources are placed. Remote after-loading machines are generally utilised, although the format of the applicators may vary. This is often an effective way of delivering radiotherapy treatment but because of the close proximity of the bladder and bowel to the radioactive sources the patient may experience some short-term side effects, the management of which is covered later.

Diathermy or laser therapy may be of some use in the management of haemoptysis or haematuria (Neal & Hoskin 1997). Sucralfate can be given orally or used topically to treat superficial bleeding (Regnard & Tempest 1992, Hoy 1993, Waller & Caroline 1996).

Kaposi's sarcoma

Kaposi's sarcoma was first described in 1872. It was known to affect elderly Ashkenazi Jewish men and is also common in Africa. It accounts for 10% of male cancers in Kenya and Uganda. It is also seen in renal transplant patients who are on long-term immunosuppressive drugs and in AIDS patients (Neal & Hoskin 1997, Souhami & Tobias 1998).

The tumour arises from the vascular endothelial cells of the skin and is seen on the limbs as purplish nodules.

In AIDS-related Kaposi's sarcoma, lesions can occur in mucous membranes, giving rise to pain, ulceration, bleeding, oedema and disfigurement (Neal & Hoskin 1997). Kaposi's sarcoma is sensitive to radiotherapy, which can be given as a single dose or possibly as a longer course of treatment in non-AIDS-related Kaposi's sarcoma.

The prognosis is poor for Kaposi's sarcoma related to AIDS. For non-AIDS-related Kaposi's sarcoma, the response to treatment lasts longer. Kaposi's sarcoma is also sensitive to some chemotherapy agents, such as anthracyclines and vinca alkaloids (Neal & Hoskin 1997, Souhami & Tobias 1998).

SIDE EFFECTS OF RADIOTHERAPY

The nursing care of patients with cancer is not just focused on the disease but on identifying and treating the side effects that patients might experience as a result of their treatment (Oliver 1988).

The side effects produced by radiotherapy occur because of the damage caused to normal cells within the path of the radiation beam. Often patients need to be reassured of this as many are concerned about side effects not associated with their treatment, such as hair loss, if the chest wall is being treated. It is always helpful to find out about any previous experience or ideas

the patient may have about radiotherapy as misconceptions can easily occur, resulting in unnecessary worry. Accurate honest information has been shown to help patients cope with the potential side effects and to give them a sense of control. Webb (1987) discusses the importance of patient teaching and how it can help the patient to be more involved with self-care. It could be argued that information-giving is the role of the medical staff, but nurses and other health care professionals are well equipped and should be able to support the patient by giving information about treatment effects, side effects and coping strategies. Patients need to understand the potential for side effects and, together with nurses, be alert for early detection. Prompt treatment of side effects by the caring team is essential (Whale 1991).

Normal cells are more able to repair damage, whereas cancer cells are more limited in their ability to repair (Kirkbride 1995, Holmes 1996b): these studies have also helped to identify normal tissues which are more sensitive to radiotherapy. In some tissues, such as the skin, bone marrow and the lining of the gastrointestinal tract, the cells have a rapid rate of replication (Holmes 1996b, Needham 1997, Souhami & Tobias 1998). Cells which divide at a slower rate will be affected by radiotherapy, but this may not become evident for some time after treatment when they start to replicate. These side effects are classed as late or chronic effects. Some of these late effects are irreversible, and patients should be made aware of them. Prompt recognition and treatment can prevent serious complications (Holmes 1996b).

Some side effects are common to radiotherapy and chemotherapy and so will be discussed at the end of the section relating to side effects from chemotherapy.

Care of site-specific side effects

Skin care

Because the epithelial cells replicate rapidly they are more sensitive to damage caused by radiation (Campbell & Lane 1996, Holmes

1996b). In their paper on developing a skin care protocol, Campbell & Lane (1996) suggest that the use of research-based skin care will remove some of the outdated practices in use. One controversial area is whether patients can wash the area being treated or not. A study conducted by Campbell & Illingworth (1992) demonstrated that there was little difference in the incidence of skin reactions between those patients who washed and those who did not. Webb (1979) points out that not washing can be distressing for patients and may be socially unacceptable.

One factor that may contribute to the development of skin reactions is friction, caused by skin surfaces rubbing together, clothes rubbing on the treated area (e.g. shirt collars) or pressure caused by position (e.g. sitting). These areas need to be closely monitored.

Patients receiving chemotherapy and radiotherapy may be more prone to developing reactions because chemotherapy can make the skin more prone to radiation damage. If a reaction does develop, the area may become reddened, like mild sunburn. This can progress from dry to moist desquamation (Campbell & Lane 1996). The skin will not repair until the treatment is complete, but prompt identification can prevent the reaction from progressing.

In patients receiving palliative radiotherapy, one would not expect to see anything more than a mild reaction, except in those patients having treatment over a 4-week period, in some head and neck cancers.

The brain

If the brain is being irradiated, the patient may experience side effects, including headaches and nausea due to raised intracranial pressure as a result of cerebral oedema caused by the tumour and the inflammatory response of the brain tissue to the radiation. Patients are generally given corticosteroids to reduce this response. Steroid-related complications such as oral candida, oedema, diabetes, dyspepsia, insomnia, and rarely, psychotic changes may occur (Regnard & Tempest 1992, Kaye 1994). These complications generally respond to a dose reduction. Analgesics and antiemetics may be administered to enhance patient comfort.

Hair loss will be a problem for the patient receiving radiotherapy to the brain; unfortunately, there is nothing that can be done to prevent this, so the patient will need support. Wigs and hairpieces may help and have a positive influence on body image but they serve as a constant reminder of the illness. Patients should be told that their hair will grow back after treatment but it may be a different colour or texture.

Head and neck

Dry eyes may become a problem but can be managed by using regular eye care and the use of eye drops, such as hypromellose. In some cases the eyes may have to be shielded to protect the lens from damage. Shields can be made of lead or tungsten, and must be inserted prior to treatment. One of the late effects from radiotherapy to this area is the formation of cataracts.

Oral care is especially important for patients receiving radiotherapy to this area because the oral mucosa is prone to damage. Palliative radiotherapy may be considered with this group of patients to relieve obstructive symptoms (Neal & Hoskin 1997). The problems related to treatment in this area include mucositis, pain, dry mouth, infection, anorexia, altered taste and psychological problems (Feber 1995). Good oral hygiene should include using a soft toothbrush and regular mouthwashes. Some over-the-counter mouthwashes contain alcohol which can dry the oral mucosa, making it more susceptible to damage. Saliva substitutes can be used to lubricate the mucous membranes (Heals 1993). High fluid intake will help to maintain lubrication. Good pain management and prompt detection and treatment of oral infections will increase comfort.

Adequate nutritional intake is important to provide the body with enough protein to enable cellular repair. This can be compromised if the patient is experiencing altered taste, anorexia or dysphagia. Effective nursing and early involvement of a dietician can help with the management of these problems. Some patients may require enteral feeding during treatment.

Chest

Oesophagitis, which can be troublesome for patients having treatment to the chest, occurs because of the rapid replication rate of the gastrointestinal mucosa. Pain can be a particular problem following intraluminal brachytherapy, because the radioactive source is close to the oesophagus. High fluid intake and an oral local anaesthetic with an alkaline or aspirin suspension will relieve pain by acting locally on the oesophageal mucosa.

Pneumonitis may occur after radiotherapy to the chest if the lungs are in the treatment field. It has an acute phase, beginning 6 weeks to 3 months after radiotherapy. Mild cases resolve but more serious cases require antibiotic treatment and steroids (Neal & Hoskin 1997). Pulmonary fibrosis and permanent respiratory compromise may result.

Pelvis

Radiotherapy to the pelvis may be used to treat cancer of the prostate, colorectal cancer, urological cancers, penile cancer and gynaecological cancers. Side effects range from early effects such as cystitis and diarrhoea, which tend to resolve in 2 to 3 weeks after completion of treatment, to late effects such as fistula formation or vaginal stenosis.

Cystitis requires prompt treatment. Infection needs to be eliminated as a cause of the cystitis. A high fluid intake needs to be encouraged: 2.5–3 litres of fluid per day is recommended. Administration of appropriate medication and monitoring of effectiveness is required.

Diarrhoea can also be a problem. Patients need to be made aware of this as it may have been a presenting symptom and cause anxiety if they are unaware that it is related to the treatment. Increased fluid intake should be encouraged to prevent dehydration. A bland low-fibre diet helps to reduce aggravation of the gastrointestinal mucosa.

If a gynaecological malignancy is being treated, fistula formation between the bowel and vagina or the bladder and vagina could be a late effect of radiotherapy. There is little that can be done to relieve this distressing effect although a surgical opinion should be sought if it does occur.

WHAT IS CHEMOTHERAPY?

Chemotherapy is the use of chemical agents that are toxic to cells (cytotoxic) aimed at eradicating or reducing the overall population of cancer cells. Unfortunately, as with radiotherapy, the drugs presently available do not act on cancer cells alone. Normal cells will also be affected, causing the patient to experience side effects. Cells which replicate rapidly are more readily affected by cytotoxic drugs (Burton 1988, Holmes 1997). This applies to both malignant and normal cells.

There are currently 40–50 cytotoxic drugs licensed to treat cancer. Pharmacology and drug administration will not be covered in this chapter but are discussed in depth by Holmes (1997), Luken & Middleton (1995) and Neal & Hoskin (1997).

Chemotherapy has proved successful in managing some childhood cancers, testicular teratoma, some lymphomas and leukaemias. There has been an increase in the use of chemotherapy as an adjuvant treatment together with surgery and/or radiotherapy, particularly in patients with breast cancer, colorectal cancer and some head and neck cancers. Studies have shown this can improve disease-free survival time in some patients (Curt & Chabner 1987 in Holmes 1997).

Palliative chemotherapy

Chemotherapy is able to destroy both the primary tumour and distant metastases (Holmes 1996c). Kaye & Levy (1997) state: 'Palliative chemotherapy may be given to patients with locally advanced or metastatic disease in order to prolong life, control symptoms or improve quality of life'. They see palliative chemotherapy as a partnership between the patient and the

vincristine and vindesine; and other drugs, such as ifosfamide, docetaxel, paclitaxel and etoposide.

Hair loss is a psychologically distressing side effect of chemotherapy. Whenery-Tedder (1997) talks of the social and psychological impact of chemotherapy-induced hair loss because of the patient's altered body image. If this happens after mutilating surgery it can prove too much to bear for some patients.

Reassurance should be given that hair will return following completion of the chemotherapy, but that the texture and colour of their hair might differ because of the effects of the drug on hair follicles. A hairpiece should be provided before hair loss occurs. Turbans and head scarves are a popular alternative.

Scalp cooling is a technique used to prevent hair loss by reducing the amount of drugs reaching the scalp (Dougherty 1996, Holmes 1997). There are a number of scalp-cooling systems in use across the country with varying degrees of success. Dougherty (1996) recommends that scalp cooling should be made available (subject to medical approval) to all patients who could benefit.

Stomatitis

A sore mouth can be caused by some chemotherapy drugs. This can range from general soreness, loss of taste, loss of papillae from the tongue, to severe painful ulceration. Stomatitis is caused because the oral mucosa replicates rapidly, making it more susceptible to the effects of chemotherapy. Some of the drugs known to cause problems are 5-fluorouracil and bleomycin.

Patient education about oral hygiene is important. An oral hygiene regimen using a soft toothbrush and regular mouthwashes can help to keep the mouth moist and clean. In addition, mouthwashes containing a topical analgesic can reduce pain. Oral assessment tools, discussed earlier in the chapter, can be beneficial.

Patients receiving chemotherapy may be prone to oral infections and the mouth can be an ideal entry point for bacteria. Corticosteroids may increase the susceptibility of the patient to developing oral candida. Treatment with any antifungal preparation will help.

Patients receiving methotrexate are particularly prone to developing mouth ulcers and may routinely be given folinic acid to encourage replication of the gastrointestinal mucosa.

Taste alteration may occur and some patients develop an aversion to certain drinks or food. Some patients also experience a metallic taste in their mouth during administration of some drugs; sucking mints or sweets may help. This can be constant or intermittent and is often distressing, so mentioning the possibility of this sensation developing can ease some of the distress experienced. The taste generally reverts to normal when chemotherapy is completed (Speechley 1989).

Peripheral neuropathy

This side effect has been seen with cisplatin and the vinca alkaloids. Although it is a late effect, presenting months after completion of treatment, it is irreversible.

Since the introduction of the taxanes, patients have been known to develop mild to moderate neuropathy with early onset. The extent of the neuropathy ranges from pins and needles to reduced mobility. This effect does appear to improve on completion of the treatment, and patients should be made aware of its possibility prior to treatment. Aston (1997) suggests that patients need to be told how to cope with this distressing symptom.

Altered bowel habits

Diarrhoea or constipation may be experienced by patients receiving chemotherapy: they are equally distressing, often causing abdominal pain and discomfort. Diarrhoea often results from the effect that chemotherapy drugs have on the gastrointestinal mucosa, and commonly occurs with the use of 5-fluorouracil, methotrexate, doxorubicin and irinotecan.

The patient may be given antidiarrhoeal medication and dietary advice, such as a bland low-fibre diet and high fluid intake – up to 3 litres of fluid a day to prevent dehydration and electrolyte imbalance.

Constipation may be a problem particularly in patients treated with vinca alkaloids, as these reduce gut motility (Holmes 1997). There may be other factors which can compound the problem, such as the use of opioid analgesics, lack of exercise and alteration in diet. Prophylactic aperients can be prescribed, together with a high-fibre diet (Holmes 1997).

Giving information to the patient at an early stage will ease some distress and anxiety caused through lack of information. It also aids early recognition of problems and enables prompt treatment, although it may cause some patients to worry.

SIDE EFFECTS COMMON TO RADIOTHERAPY AND CHEMOTHERAPY
Nausea and vomiting

Nausea and vomiting are two distressing side effects related to radiotherapy and chemotherapy. With radiotherapy they may be related to the area or the duration of treatment. The byproducts of cell breakdown, urea and creatinine, are normally toxic in large amounts. Large numbers of cells are being broken down as a result of treatment. The toxins produced will be detected in the blood by the chemoreceptor trigger zone and a response initiated. These mechanisms are discussed more fully by Williams (1994) and Holmes (1997).

Oliver et al (1997) state: 'It is now possible to control the distressing adverse effects of chemotherapy. Very potent antiemetics have rendered even the most emetogenic regimens controllable'. With the introduction of drugs such as 5-HT$_3$ antagonists this has increased the number of drugs available to help in the management of nausea and vomiting.

There are a number of factors that can induce nausea and vomiting (Williams 1994), and others that can predispose a person to be more likely to develop nausea and vomiting, such as motion sickness (Adams 1993). Good assessment of the patient will help ensure appropriate prescribing of antiemetic drugs and reduce the incidence of this side effect.

It is helpful to understand the mechanisms involved in producing this response, which in turn aids more appropriate prescribing of antiemetics (Williams 1994). Williams (1994) states: 'Psychologically, uncontrolled nausea and vomiting may well cause anxiety and distress to patients, their relatives and friends'.

Quinton (1998) says that: 'maintaining adequate control of nausea and vomiting can preserve the quality of an individual's life and enable patients and their families to endure what can be a demanding courses of chemotherapy'.

Anticipatory nausea and vomiting is difficult to manage and occurs in patients who have previously had aggressive chemotherapy. Lorazepam can be used, as it is an anxiolytic. Patients may forget the experience of vomiting.

Hypnotherapy can be used to help in the management of anticipatory nausea and vomiting by offering the patient a sense of control (Stein 1996). Other complementary measures such as pressure bands are described by Stannard (1989). Distraction or acupuncture have also been used with some success.

Bone marrow depression

This can present as anaemia, leucopenia and thrombocytopenia. Myelosuppression can be caused by both radiotherapy or chemotherapy; the presenting signs and care of the patient are similar, regardless of the cause.

With radiotherapy the development and extent of myelosuppression depends on the extent of bone marrow in the treatment field (Holmes 1996a). The structure of the bone marrow may be permanently altered, leaving the patient compromised (Holmes 1996a).

Regular monitoring of the blood count may be carried out as a high red blood count is beneficial during treatment. It helps oxygenate the cancer cells, which potentiates the damaging affect of radiation.

Luken & Middleton (1995) and Stein (1996) point out that the myelosuppression caused by chemotherapy is the most common dose-limiting toxicity and is potentially fatal. A degree of myelosuppression is produced by all chemotherapy

CASE STUDY 5.1

INTRODUCTION

Palliative care is a programme of active, compassionate care which is primarily directed towards improving the quality of life. It is a discipline with its own growing research and knowledge base, and a specific set of skills aimed at symptom control and psychological support. Palliative care allows explicit goals for therapy and informed choices for patients. All the family is affected by the chronic illness of one member and so palliative care services involve the whole family as the unit of care. Holistic care for both patient and family is delivered by an interdisciplinary team (Hanson & Cullihall 1996). This study is unusual because of the palliative measures taken to alleviate difficult symptoms of oesophageal and secondary pyloric carcinoma – using modern invasive techniques. The team faced many difficulties, supporting the patient and his family through many disappointments. This time was also emotionally and physically demanding for those who cared for the patient. The study will make clear why modern techniques to prolong and sustain life in the terminally ill should be used despite negative attitudes expressed by others. A combination of team effort and minimally invasive techniques brought comfort and dignity to the patient and his family.

Patient history

Dave, a 56-year-old man, was diagnosed with oesophageal carcinoma. He lived with his loving wife, Sylvia. His only daughter was married but remained close to her father. Seven months ago, an oesophagectomy was performed. The stomach was pulled into the right thoracic cavity and the upper part of the oesophagus was joined to the immobilised stomach and duodenum. A node dissection was performed at surgery. Dave received a course of radiotherapy soon after his surgical recovery. He was re-admitted 4 months later because of epigastric pain and occasional nausea and vomiting. An oesophagogastroduodenostomy (OGD) examination 2 days later revealed recurrent cancer obstructing the gastric pylorus. Abdominal ultrasound showed liver metastases, and a chest X-ray demonstrated chest abnormalities.

On admission Dave was told about the possible recurrence and advancement of his disease and that his cancer was incurable. Dave and Sylvia were extremely anxious. Dave had not retired and they had made many plans, thinking the initial surgery had been successful. Their first grandchild would soon be born.

Primary nursing was used to ensure continuity in nursing care throughout Dave's stay. His nursing care was organised using the Roper et al (1980) model of nursing. The surgical team and palliative care teams worked together to care for Dave and his family. The primary nurse ensured that Sylvia was an integral part of his care. Care was planned around a usual daily routine, while Dave was in hospital. Most of his subsequent care took place in a hospice, which helped ease the family's distress. Dave's initial aim was to `get over this set-back'. He wanted to live at home within the surroundings he and Sylvia had worked hard for over the years. Dave never suffered from ill health, until he complained of difficulty in swallowing 4 months before his operation. Sadly, his disease had now spread, and Dave and Sylvia knew that time together was the only thing valuable during this difficult journey towards death from an unwanted disease.

Oesophageal cancer

Oesophageal cancer is commoner in males, with a male to female ratio of about 2:1, and usually occurs in individuals over 50 years of age (Belcher 1992). In the United Kingdom it has become more prevalent in the last 10 years. There is much evidence to say it is related to excessive alcohol and tobacco smoking, as well as to nutritional deficiencies and environmental carcinogens (Souhami & Tobias 1998).

Dysphagia is the commonest symptom and is almost always accompanied by weight loss, often amounting to 10% or more of body weight. Recent evidence strongly supports the view that adenocarcinoma of the oesophagus is rising in incidence (Powel & McConkey 1990). Excision is the treatment of choice in patients who are generally fit and with no evidence of distant metastases. It is important to determine the extent of the lesion before definitive surgery. There is no evidence that preoperative radiotherapy influences recovery from the resection, operative mortality or overall survival (Earlam & Cunha-Melo 1980).

Dave's operation employed a technique using mobilised stomach above the diaphragm (Fig. 5.4) as a means of reconstruction. This is an extensive operation and has a high risk of mortality. Surgical complications such as oesophageal stricture, anastomotic leak – resulting in mediastinitis, pneumonitis and septicaemia – can be fatal (Souhami & Tobias 1998).

With intensive nursing, Dave's surgery and recovery was successful without complications. He was discharged home until his present re-admission with new symptoms and pain.

ISSUES REQUIRING CARE

Pain

Dave was experiencing epigastric pain, which became worse with episodes of nausea. It was difficult to know if it was tumour pain or discomfort caused by the nausea. For most patients physical pain is one of the greatest fears associated with cancer. Dave was afraid of morphine because of his experience when recovering from his surgery. He had experienced hallucinations and was reluctant to take any medication. Although this is understandable, especially in responding as a nurse to a particular pain problem, the temptation may be to focus on

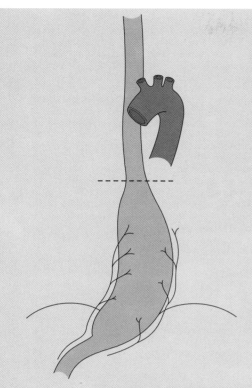

Figure 5.4 Surgery for oesophageal cancer, showing gastric mobilisation and pull-through for carcinoma of the lower third, reprinted with kind permission of Blackwell Science Ltd.

that symptom alone. The patient must be allowed to identify his problems and interventions should honour the value of the patient's perceptions (Davies & Oberle 1990).

Pain assessment

Dave was allowed to talk about his fears about pain and to tell his story as a means of assessment. He looked pale and anxious. He talked about his original diagnosis and his and his family's hopes following the surgery. The pain seemed to indicate to Dave and his wife that the cancer had returned and they were frightened. They felt the possibility of metastatic spread had not been made clear to them at the time of his first operation. They both had ambivalent feelings towards medical staff and health care professionals. These feelings faded with careful handling, honesty and truth. Although Dave's general practitioner had asked for an urgent referral to the consultant he waited 4 weeks for admission. Despite the informality of the information gathering, the responses were sorted into pain concepts, so that appropriate resources could be utilised. Dave loved life: he was looking forward to having grandchildren. He now felt he

would never work again or drive a car and that, ultimately, this was the end.

It was decided to discuss Dave's fears of morphine with medical staff before choosing an appropriate analgesic. At this point a pain and symptom chart was introduced, using a new chart piloted by the ward, combining pain and associated symptoms on one chart. This was used to record when Dave admitted to having pain or was observed and assessed as having pain and when analgesics were administered. There is a need for simple, efficient and valid assessment tools that can provide rapid evaluation in clinical settings of the major aspects of pain experienced by cancer patients (Foley 1982).

In view of Dave's nausea and the unsuitability of oral analgesics, it was decided to use 150 mg tramadol administered subcutaneously via a 24-hour syringe driver. Tramadol is a safe and effective agent introduced in the late 1970s to alleviate cancer pain. Its efficacy appears to be equivalent to that of morphine but is dose-dependent. It causes less constipation or respiratory depression. It causes weak activation of both central pain and inhibitory mechanisms in the opioid receptors as well as the descending mono-aminergic system (Budd 1995). Initially, tramadol did not control Dave's pain, so the dose was increased.

Dave experienced anxiety and depression as a result of his illness and altered body image. Both these emotions are likely to exacerbate his pain symptoms. Saunders (1990) described somatic and psychological experience of pain as 'total pain'. It is also directly related to the pain gate theory (Melzack & Wall 1965), and the role of the limbic system in which anxiety and depression serve to open the gate to varying degrees, thus heightening pain perception. It was important for the nurses to provide a supportive environment for Dave and his family.

Nausea

Dave was experiencing nausea on admission which was problematic; a gastroscopy revealed the recurrence of cancer at the pylorus of the immobilised stomach. The lumen from the pylorus had a stricture into the duodenum caused by the tumour, thus preventing the passage of food or fluids (Fig. 5.5a).

A nasogastric tube had been inserted. It was allowed to drain freely and aspirated every 2 hours to keep the stomach empty. Intravenous therapy was started to establish and maintain a fluid intake of 3 litres in 24 hours.

In the hospice, fluids were given subcutaneously (hypodermoclysis). Hypodermoclysis is defined as the infusion of a solution into the subcutaneous tissue to supply the patient with a continuous and sufficient amount of fluid, electrolytes or nutrients (Urdang 1983). This is an easy and effective way to administer fluids.

Dave was kept informed about his treatment and told the findings of the gastroscopy by the surgeon. Surgical treatment to restore the continuity of the

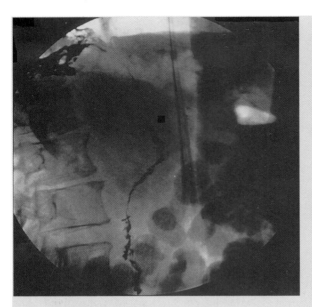

Figure 5.5a X-ray showing the stricture of pylorus, with kind permission of South Tyneside District Hospital.

lumen could not be considered and other palliative treatments such as radiotherapy and chemotherapy were not an option at this stage. This meant that Dave would continue like this and die soon.

Percutaneous gastroscopy (also known as venting gastroscopy) is often a last resort. The stomach drains continuously via a tube placed through the abdomen into the stomach. This allows the patient to drink without vomiting, as the fluids drain into a collecting bag (Ashby et al 1991). For Dave, the option of percutaneous gastroscopy was also impossible as his stomach was in his chest.

It was decided that 150 mg cyclizine would be given concurrently with tramadol via the subcutaneous route to control Dave's nausea. Cyclizine is an antihistamine with added anticholinergic activity. This drug was chosen as symptoms of bowel obstruction may be mediated by partly vagal afferent fibres (*Mosby Drug Reference* 1994).

Once the nausea and pain were relieved Dave slept for long periods over night. Sylvia was feeling guilty because he was in hospital and he wanted to be at home with his family. He reconciled himself that he was in an environment where additional support was available 24 hours a day should his symptoms return. Sylvia was always in a guilt dilemma and often needed reassurance from nursing staff that Dave was in the best place. Sylvia's own sleep pattern varied and as time moved on she began to look tired and thin.

The next day after careful consideration and discussion with a radiologist, the team decided that the only option was to try an expansile

metal stent implanted in the pyloric stricture to open up the lumen of the bowel. This would alleviate Dave's nausea and he would be able to manage oral medications and a modified liquid diet. He would not need intravenous fluids or nasogastric aspiration. This procedure is not without risks. Incorrect dilatation of the lumen during stent insertion carries the risk of bowel perforation. The recent use of expansile metallic stents had demonstrated an improved survival rate in patients like Dave. He felt at ease with this solution. He agreed to the procedure and the stent arrived within 2 days. During this time Dave's pain and symptoms were controlled. Preliminary X-rays were taken using a contrast opaque solution, instilled via the nasogastric tube. The X-rays enabled the length of the stricture to be measured, and allowed assessment of the extent of the stenosis and a decision on the position of the stent.

Metallic stent insertion
Normally an oesophageal expansile stent is never used in the pylorus and duodenum, because the peristaltic movement in this part of the bowel may dislodge the stent. Dave consented for the procedure, which took place in the radiology department using an image intensifier. When Dave was positioned on the table (supine), an electrocardiograph (ECG) monitor was attached and oximetry attached by ear probe to measure oxygen saturation (normal value > 92–94%). Oxygen was given via a nasal cannula throughout and his blood pressure was measured pre- and post-sedation with midazolam (increments of 2 mg given every 3 minutes if required). A nurse monitored his airway and vital signs throughout the procedure.

Insertion technique
1. A contrast solution was instilled via the nasogastric tube into the pylorus and stomach; at that time the head end of the table was raised.
2. No contrast solution was seen to enter the duodenum so a guidewire was passed into the stomach and pushed with some force through the stricture,
3. Dilators were threaded one at a time over the guidewire, to dilate the stricture. At one point, contrast was seen to trickle into the duodenum, indicating a passage could be made.
4. After dilatation to the satisfaction of the radiologist, a special inflatable balloon dilator was threaded over the guidewire. The balloon could only be inflated to a pre-set pressure so as not to rupture the duodenum or pylorus. Only if a final dilatation was successful and satisfactory to the radiologist would the stent be considered.
5. The stent was now threaded over the guidewire encased within its gelatine covering. It proved very difficult to place, taking almost 2 hours, needing removal and re-insertion and encountering many problems. The procedure was almost abandoned because of the difficulties. Another attempt was made, with extra pressure pushing the stent into the pylorus and duodenum; it was painful for Dave so he was given 50 mg pethidine intravenously with

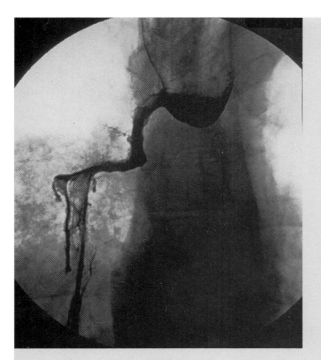

Figure 5.5b X-ray showing the stent insertion and free-flowing contrast solution through the completely opened stent, with kind permission of South Tyneside District Hospital.

2 mg of midazolam. Finally, the stent was in position the cover was removed, allowing the holding gel to dissolve and the stent to expand to its maximum size.

6. The stent was expanded internally by the insertion of the balloon dilator, to dilate the internal diameter to 12 mm. This would ensure that the whole stent would remain open.

7. More contrast solution was instilled, via the nasogastric tube. This showed that there was free flow through the stent and demonstrated a complete and successful procedure (Fig. 5.5b).

Dave returned to the ward for observation, and he awoke from sedation to hear the news of a successful positioning of the stent with good function.

The position and function of the stent was re-checked the next day and free clear oral fluids were commenced. It was checked again 5 days later; the extent of expansion was confirmed by X-ray (Fig. 5.5c).

Nutrition
The stent did not interfere with peristalsis but the pylorus could only cope with fluids. Dave's whole dietary intake was monitored and controlled by the dietician who provided a high-protein, high-calorie

diet. Medication was given in syrup form until his condition deteriorated, then a syringe driver was used to administer analgesia continuously.

Pain revisited
As Dave's pain increased there was no alternative but to give morphine, as morphine slow release sachets (MST) in liquid form. The doctor prescribed MST, 30 mg 12 hourly, and 10 mg of oral morphine solution for breakthrough pain. He was also prescribed a laxative daily, to prevent constipation, and haloperidol subcutaneously at night, to alleviate nausea associated with the morphine. Dave never experienced hallucinations and his pain was well controlled.

The analgesic protocol enabled the registered nurse to respond promptly to Dave's pain without delay or needing to refer to a doctor each time Dave was in pain. Specifically, opioids are given by the clock (Latham 1991).

As Dave weakened, his medications were altered. Diamorphine replaced the MST and methotrimeprazine, 30 mg over 24 hours, was given via a syringe driver to relieve nausea. He responded well as methotrimeprazine (Nozinan) is an antipsychotic drug which has anxiolytic and antiemetic properties and it is also a sedative (*Guys Drug Reference* 1994). It can be increased to 250 mg in 24 hours and can potentiate the action of diamorphine, causing further sedation.

Dave continued to weaken and gradually became unconscious. He died later that night surrounded by his family, 4 months after stent placement.

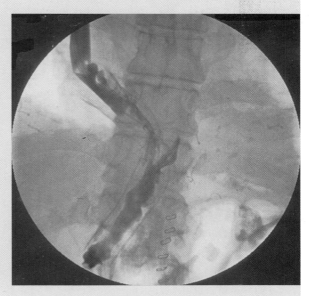

Figure 5.5c Check X-ray 5 days following insertion of the stent, with kind permission of South Tyneside District Hospital.

CONCLUSION

Palliative treatments allowed greater freedom, a relatively pain-free existence and the vomiting never returned. Dave was able to go home occasionally at weekends to be with his family before his condition deteriorated. At Christmas, everyone felt guilty tucking into Christmas dinner, while Dave had a strained soup and Fresubin, a supplementary feed. He did manage some alcohol: he loved Guinness. Open communication with Dave and his family helped throughout the few months that he had left. They were allowed to make informed choices regarding his care. The metallic stent was a great aid to his palliation, allowing Dave to die with dignity, in control and with no vomiting, pain or discomfort.

Without the stent, his life would have been shorter and possibly unbearable. The nursing staff played a valuable role as part of the palliative care team helping to alleviate Dave's anxiety and restlessness and to control his pain and nausea. This allowed him to have quality time to spend with his family.

REFERENCES

Adams L 1993 Managing chemotherapy-induced nausea and vomiting. Professional Nurse 9(2): 91–94

Ashby M A, Game P A, Devitt P et al 1991 Percutaneous gastrostomy as venting procedure in palliative care. Palliative Medicine 5: 147–150

Aston V 1997 Patient management and docetaxel. International Journal of Palliative Nursing 3(3): 175–178

Belcher E A 1992 Cancer nursing. Mosby Year Book, St. Louis

Budd K 1995 Tramadol – A step towards the ideal analgesia. European Journal of Palliative Care 2(2): 56–60

Burton S 1988 Cytotoxic drugs. Professional Nurse 3(11): 447–452

Calvert H, McElwain T 1988 The role of chemotherapy. In: Pritchard P (ed.) Oncology for nurses and health care professionals, 2nd edn. Vol 1, Pathology, diagnosis and treatment. Harper and Row, Beaconsfield, p. 298

Campbell I, Illingworth M 1992 Can patients wash during radiotherapy to the breast or chest wall? – A randomised controlled trial. Clinical Oncology 4: 78–82

Campbell J, Lane M A 1996 Developing a skin care protocol in radiotherapy. Professional Nurse 12(2): 105–108

Coleman R E 1996a Oncological emergencies. In: Hancock B W (ed.) Cancer care in the community. Radcliffe Medical Press, Oxford, p. 94

Coleman R E 1996b Cancer of the female genital tract. In: Hancock B W (ed.) Cancer care in the hospital. Radcliffe Medical Press, Oxford, p. 108

Coleman R E 1996c Cancer of the male genital tract. In: Hancock B W (ed.) Cancer care in the hospital. Radcliffe Medical Press, Oxford, p. 120

Coleman R E and Hancock B W 1996 Cytotoxic chemotherapy: principles and practice. In: Hancock B W (ed.) Cancer care in the hospital. Radcliffe Medical Press, Oxford, p. 49

Copp K 1991 Nursing patients having radiotherapy. In: Borley D (ed.) Oncology for nurses and health care professionals, Vol 3. Harper and Row, London, p. 38

Davies B, Oberle K 1990 Dimensions of the supportive role of the nurse in palliative care. Oncology Nursing Forum 17: 87–94

Day J 1998 Alleviating bone pain using strontium therapy. Professional Nurse 14(4): 263–266

Dougherty L 1996 Scalp cooling to prevent hair loss in chemotherapy. Professional Nurse 11(8): 507–509

Earlam R, Cunha-Melo J R 1980 Oesophageal squamous cell carcinoma. British Journal of Surgery 67: 381–390

Feber T 1995 Mouth care for patients receiving oral irradiation. Professional Nurse 10(10): 666–670

Fleisch H 1995 Bisphosphonates in bone disease – from the laboratory to the patient, 2nd edn. The Parthenon Publishing Group, London

Foley K M 1982 Clinical assessment of pain. Acta Anaesthesiologica Scandinavica (Suppl) 74: 91–96. In: Doyle D, Hanks G, Macdonald N (eds) Oxford textbook of palliative medicine. Oxford University Press, Oxford, 1994, p. 155

Green P, Kinghorn S 1995 Radiotherapy. In: David J (ed.) Cancer care prevention, treatment and palliation. Chapman and Hall, London, p. 113

Griffiths A and Beaver K 1997 Quality of life during high dose chemotherapy for breast cancer. International Journal of Palliative Nursing 3(3): 138–144

Guys Drug Reference 1994 Nursing drug reference, 2nd edn, Joshua A, King T (eds). Mosby-Year Book Europe Ltd, London

Hancock B W, Robinson M H, Rees R C 1996 Other treatments. In: Hancock B W (ed.) Cancer care in the hospital. Radcliffe Medical Press, Oxford, p. 67

Hanson E J, Cullihall K 1996 Images of palliative nursing care. Journal of Palliative Care 11(3): 35–39

Heals D 1993 A key to well being: oral hygiene in patients with advanced cancer. Professional Nurse 8(6): 391–398

Heyse-Moore L 1993 Symptom control – respiratory symptoms. In: Saunders C, Sykes N (eds) The management of terminal malignant disease. Edward Arnold, London, p. 76

Holmes S 1996a Radiotherapy – A guide for practice, 2nd edn. Asset Books, Surrey

Holmes S 1996b Making sense of radiotherapy: curative and palliative. Nursing Times 92(23): 32–33

Holmes S 1996c Making sense of cancer chemotherapy. Nursing Times 92(36): 42–43

Holmes S 1997 Cancer chemotherapy – a guide for practice, 2nd edn. Asset Books, Surrey

Hoskin P 1994 Changing trends in palliative radiotherapy. In: Tobias J S, Thomas P R M (eds) Current radiation oncology, Vol. 1. Edward Arnold, London

Hoy A 1993 Symptom control – other symptom challenges. In: Saunders C, Sykes N (eds) The management of terminal malignant disease. Edward Arnold, London, p. 160

Kaye P 1994 A–Z pocketbook of symptom control. EPL Publications, Northampton

Kaye P, Levy D 1997 Palliative chemotherapy. In: Kaye P (ed.) Tutorials in palliative medicine. EPL Publications, Northampton, p. 39

Kirkbride P 1995 The role of radiation therapy in palliative care. Journal of Palliative Care 11(1): 19–26

Latham J 1991 Pain control, 2nd edn. Austen Cornish Publishers, London

Ling J 1997 Clinical trials, palliative care and the research nurse. International Journal of Palliative Nursing 3(4): 192–195

Luken J, Middleton J 1995 Chemotherapy and the administration of cytotoxic drugs into established lines. In: David J (ed.) Cancer care prevention, treatment and palliation. Chapman and Hall, London, p. 77

Melzack R, Wall P 1965 The challenge of pain. Penguin, England

Moody M, Grocott P 1993 Let us extend our knowledge base: assessment and management of fungating malignant wounds. Professional Nurse 8(9): 586–590

Moore J 1995 Biological and hormonal therapy. In: David J (ed.) Cancer care prevention, treatment and palliation. Chapman and Hall, London, p. 174

Mosby Drug Reference, Guys Hospital 1994. Mosby, St Louis

Neal A J, Hoskin P J 1997 Clinical oncology: basic principles and practice, 2nd edn. Arnold, London

Needham P 1997 Palliative radiotherapy. In: Kaye P (ed.) Tutorials in palliative medicine. EPL Publications, Northampton, p. 17

O'Brien T 1993 Symptom control – pain. In: Saunders C, Sykes N (eds) The management of terminal malignant disease. Edward Arnold, London, p. 33

Oliver G 1988 Radiotherapy. In: Tschudin V (ed.) Nursing the patient with cancer. Prentice Hall, London

Oliver G, McIllmurray M, Ashton V, Harding S, Donovan G 1997 Active palliative anti-cancer therapy. International Journal of Palliative Nursing 3(4): 232–237

Powel J M, McConkey C C 1990 Increasing incidence of adenocarcinoma of the gastric cardia and adjacent sites. British Journal of Cancer 62: 440–443

Quinton D 1998 Anticipatory nausea and vomiting in chemotherapy. Professional Nurse 13(10): 663–666

Regnard C F B, Tempest S 1992 A guide to symptom relief in advanced cancer, 3rd edn. Haigh and Hochland, Manchester

Richardson A 1995 Fatigue in cancer patients: a review of the literature. European Journal of Cancer Care 4: 20–32

Richardson J 1989 Bone metastases. Professional Nurse 4(9): 438–442

Robinson M H, Coleman R E 1996 Treatment of cancer. In: Hancock B (ed.) Cancer care in the community. Radcliffe Medical Press, Oxford, p. 38

Roper N, Logan W W, Tierney A J 1980 Learning to use the nursing process. Churchill Livingstone, Edinburgh

Saunders C 1990 Hospice and palliative care – an interdisciplinary approach. Edward Arnold, London

Smith A M 1993 Symptom control – fractures. In: Saunders C, Sykes N (eds) The management of terminal malignant disease. Edward Arnold, London, p. 149

Snape D, Robinson A 1996 Radiotherapy. In: Tschudin V (ed.) Nursing the patient with cancer, 2nd edn. Prentice Hall, Hertfordshire, p. 61

Souhami R, Tobias J 1998 Cancer and its management, 3rd edn. Blackwell Science Ltd, Oxford

Speechley V 1989 Nursing patients having chemotherapy. In: Borley D (ed.) Oncology for nurses and health care professionals. Vol. 3 Cancer nursing. Harper and Row, London, p. 74

Stannard D 1989 Pressure prevents nausea. Nursing Times 85(4): 33–34

Stein P 1996 Chemotherapy. In: Tschudin V (ed.) Nursing the patient with cancer, 2nd edn. Prentice Hall, Hertfordshire, p. 78

Stone P, Richards M, Hardy J 1998 Review fatigue in patients with cancer. European Journal of Cancer Care 34(11): 1670–1676

Twycross R 1997 Symptom management in advanced cancer, 2nd edn. Radcliffe Medical Press, Oxon

Urdang L 1983 Mosby medical and nursing dictionary. Mosby, London

Waller A, Caroline N L 1996 Handbook of palliative care in cancer. Butterworth-Heinemann, Newton

Watkinson A F, Adam A (eds) 1996 Interventional radiology – a practical guide. Radcliffe Medical Press, London

Webb P 1979 Nursing care of patient undergoing treatment by teletherapy. In: Tiffany R (ed.) Cancer nursing – radiotherapy. Faber and Faber, London, p. 78

Webb P 1987 Patient education. Nursing 20: 748, 750

Whale Z 1991 A threat to femininity? Minimising side effects in pelvic irradiation. Professional Nurse 6(6): 309–311

Whenery-Tedder M 1997 A positive approach to chemotherapy. Nursing Times 93(23): 52–53

Williams C 1994 Causes and management of nausea and vomiting. Nursing Times 90(44): 38–41

6

Spirituality: the professionals' and the patients' perspectives

Christine Searle

INTRODUCTION

The sure thing about life is that we die, and in this chapter I would like you to consider whether sufficient resources or time is given to consider the role of those charged with patient care in identifying and responding to the spiritual needs of patients as they come to terms with dying.

My experience of caring for and supporting the dying patient is based on many years working as a nurse in the community and hospice. Recognising and facilitating the spiritual needs of the dying patient greatly eases the pain that death causes for all concerned.

This chapter reviews spirituality from a medical, nursing and philosophical and theological perspective. From this, the discussion will explore the strengths and weaknesses of using a model of transition which may enable health care professionals to respond to patients' spiritual conflict. A reflective scenario of a palliative care patient called Anne is used to support and illuminate the discussion. A research project conducted by Searle et al (1999), which illustrates how focus groups can help patients identify their spiritual pain, is discussed. In conclusion, the chapter illustrates the overall discussion about spirituality and the perception of palliative care patients, professionals and carers.

Palliative care professes to deliver care based on Cicely Saunders' philosophy of holistic care, which addresses the physical, psychological and spiritual needs of patients.

In a multidisciplinary setting it can be demonstrated that physical and social needs can be defused and met by medical, nursing, paramedic and social work. Grey (1994) substantiates that these components are reasonably clear and understood, while the spiritual domain is less easily defined. This can result in a fragmented approach and, perhaps, a failing to address the spiritual pain, conflict and needs of patients within the palliative care.

An analysis of spiritual pain is difficult to produce; its meaning is diverse and amorphous because it encompasses individual belief, values and meaning of life. Hall (1997) criticises research methods that involve the use of charts, lists and structured interviews or questionnaires. She criticises scales and abstract theories, suggesting that they give false reassurance about our knowledge. Hall cautions that theories can block intuition and routinise care.

Watson (1996) talks about a contemporary crisis of caring in the wake of advances in medical science and technology. She identifies an oppressed human spirit in our modern health care system. This has serious implications for the health care of patients within a palliative care setting. These patients will undoubtedly be experiencing loss, fear, despair and may well be searching, perhaps for the first time, for a meaning and purpose to their existence.

The implications for the health care professional is that there is a profound professional duty to ensure that spiritual pain, conflict and needs are dealt with from the perception of the patient by whoever the patient chooses. This requires multi-professional palliative care to be collaborative and individual case study based. It requires a common core understanding of the difference between spiritual needs and religious needs by each member of the multidisciplinary team, including clerics and religious representatives.

A clear understanding of roles and best practice relating to spirituality should enable patients to identify and understand their spirituality, and in turn, assist them in choosing the person or means to enable them to spiritually care for themselves and their significant others.

THE MEDICAL PERSPECTIVE

McKee & Chappel (1992) imply that spirituality is not often addressed in medical practice. They suggest personal discomfort with the subject and concern about imposing one's own beliefs on patients could be the reason, or the belief that medicine is essentially a science and that spirituality is a tangible and abstract concept.

They cite Barnard (1983) as focusing on four areas within religion and medicine:

- the meaning of health and illness
- the relation of health to other human values
- attitudes towards the aged, incurable and weak
- attitudes towards nature.

It is impossible for all individuals to share the same beliefs, but in health care it is essential that we understand and respect individual beliefs. McKee and Chappel acknowledge the fact that spirituality is not provable or quantifiable. They recommend that integrated medical and hospital clergy training may add to a dimension in spiritual health care.

Cassell (1982) implies that suffering can be a result of disease but also that modern medicine can be the cause of suffering. This paradox, he suggests, has implications for how doctors view the meaning or interpretation of illness for the patient. He suggests that the advance in medical science welcomed the Cartesian dualism of mind–body split and as a result passed the spiritual realms to the Church. It could be viewed that this 'buck passing' has contributed to the deficit of professional responsibility for spiritual care. He compares and contrasts different issues of suffering as a result of pain and concurs that when patients know the reason for their pain, the pain is more acceptable and tolerated. He highlights the significance of personal meaning and acknowledges that suffering has a bodily emotional and spiritual transcendent meaning. However, he emphasises that medical advances continue to enlighten us about the interpretation of suffering.

Alderidge (1991) recognises the importance of 'making sense' of the illness experience for patients and suggests there is a search for meaning in the face of loss and suffering. This time of chaos for the patient clearly calls for assessing and addressing the spirituality of patients. He contends that the issues underpinning the definition of health and healing are challenging in this age when the Church and medicine are undergoing continual transformation.

Domminian (1983) acknowledges the connection between doctors and patients which requires trust, faith and hope, and suggests that the role of the doctor is to transform the ordinary into the extraordinary – the human into the divine. He recognises that this will be challenged by those who say that hope and trust are about being human (rather than divine). However, he suggests that these are human experiences: to live them fully requires a degree of persistent motivation relating to a power beyond human existence.

He identifies healing as entailing physical, emotional and spiritual integrity:

- the physical can be addressed by surgery or therapeutic intervention
- the emotional can be changed by transforming the psyche
- the spirit can be changed by bringing a person in touch with ultimate values and the purpose of living.

He implies that illness can be a powerful source of change and that the doctor has to recognise the spiritual reserves of the patient. This could be an overt faith in God or may, in the absence of God, take the form of persistent determination, peace, faith in life, endurance, hope, optimism and a certainty that death is not the end. He recommends collaborative understanding of spiritual care, instead of going separate ways and recognising the common predicament that is the ultimate value of the transcendental or 'going beyond'.

Mathers (1976) focused on the concept of personal identity needs, but suggested that medi-cine, theology and social sciences tend to view human nature with detachment.

Millard (1976) suggests that anxiety relates to a sense of 'being' and, therefore, is heightened by the threat of 'non-being'. He describes spiritual anxiety as the anxiety of meaningless and emptiness and suggests that the threat of biological extinction and complete loss of self is the main cause of spiritual anxiety. In palliative care, anxiety is a core symptom which accompanies the patient from the self-suspicion of illness to diagnosis and prognosis. While anxiety is acknowledged by patient, relatives and professionals, it is often not related to spirituality.

Maughans (1996) highlights the fact that there is little recent literature relating to the medical involvement of spiritual care. He recommends that health care professionals:

- consider spirituality as a potentially important component of every patient's well-being
- consider addressing spirituality with patients early and often; although a spiritual history can be obtained in a single patient encounter
- respect the patient's autonomy and privacy of spiritual beliefs and practices: avoid overt projection of your private belief system onto others
- identify the spiritual resources in your community and use them appropriately
- reflect on your own spirituality and how it impacts on your concept of self, your relationships and practice.

This comprehensive contemplation of spirituality, he suggests, aids exploration of this potentially vital area of patient care.

Atkinson (1993) challenges whether illness needs to have a meaning. She implies that using adjectives such as 'suffer' can medicalise patient care and patients may miss the opportunity to focus on positive times or points of their lives when they do not suffer. There is a fine line or grey area between the need for meaning to illness and the existence of illness. Labelling people as victims or sufferers can have disadvantages. Not exploring the meaning of the illness for the patient could have grave implications for unmanaged spiritual pain.

Cobb (1997) infers that despite a general decline in religious practice it cannot be assumed that people have no beliefs or that they have lost their spiritual dimension. Indeed, he suggests that beliefs and faith are a psychological necessity for living – making sense of reality and finding meaning. Palliative care aspires to making spiritual care part of total care and, therefore, concerns all staff. He warns, however, that it can be difficult to distinguish spiritual care from emotional care and it may lose its focus and value when routinely included with organised care.

It is the assumption made by some health care professionals that if the box indicating the patient's religion is ticked, then spirituality has been addressed; thus, assumptions can be made for connivance or for embarrassment or awkwardness within the health care professional. Something may challenge or threaten their own moral integrity: justification to self that 'it's not my job, it's the job of the chaplain'. Another assumption is that the clergy can help. Recent research (Searle et al 1999) suggests that the chaplain or priest can in fact sometimes serve to aggravate spiritual distress, which then remains unrelieved and unsupported.

THE NURSING PERSPECTIVE

The nursing literature offers a wide variety of definitions of spirituality. There is for the most part an agreement that there is ambiguity and confusion about the relationship between spirituality and conventional religious belief systems.

Synonymy between religion and spirituality may not always be appropriate, but as Narayanasamy (1993) and Dyson et al (1997) imply, individuals often see a relationship between spirituality and religion. This is often compounded by the fact that many of the studies which have explored spirituality use subjects who hold profound Christian beliefs.

Boutell & Bozett (1990), Narayanasamy (1993), Ross (1994), Turner (1996), McSherry (1996) and Martsolf & Mickley (1998) all emphasise a gap in nurse education with regard to a lack of preparation and attention to spirituality in nursing which is very concerning. According to Ross (1994), spiritual care should be a nursing responsibility and not an optional extra.

Turner (1996) implies that nurses are losing the opportunity to attend to spiritual needs in patients as a result of increased pressure to describe and justify nursing intervention. McGrath (1999) highlights the difficulties in collating evidence about spirituality management suggesting that to date most of our understanding has evolved from 'anecdotal evidence from charismatic hospice leaders' (McGrath 1999, p. 3). Goddard (1995) considers the need for empirical concerns on the components of spirituality and urges its integration into nursing curricular. The author feels that this lack of consensus probably results from the ambiguity of the term and 'all this talk, no action', which enables health care professionals to avoid responsibility as far as spiritual care is concerned. While we can usually get away with this in the general health care setting, palliative care demands more. As Reed (1991) implies, the spiritual perspective is greater in those who are aware of the terminal potential of their disease and that people with cancer have a mortality awareness that brings their spiritual and psychological needs to the foreground. The author suggests that despite the technological and scientific emphasis on care, nurses have a unique and intimate relationship with patients which should enable them to address spiritual conflict or pain. She recommends that this should begin with self-exploration. As the expression suggests, this should not require sophisticated equipment or documentation or even involve a religious person and/or system. However, a key worker within a palliative care interdisciplinary team could focus on enabling the patient to relax and to develop self-awareness and relaxation through techniques such as breathing exercises, aromatherapy, reflexology, music and art appreciation. Also, as Burnard (1993) suggests, attributes such as genuineness, empathy, non-judgemental and unconditional positive regard can help patients uncomplicate their thoughts and feelings within a therapeutic dialogue.

McSherry (1996) raises concern about the misconception and ambiguity relating to spiritual and religious needs and implies that nursing education is failing to address this issue.

THEOLOGICAL AND PHILOSOPHICAL PERSPECTIVE

To identify spiritual pain we need to understand its origins. Mickley & Sochen Belcher (1992) define religiousness as 'personal meaning that individuals attach to a particular set of beliefs, values, rules of conduct and rituals'. They suggest that spiritual well-being is multidimensional but focuses on two main issues, namely existential and religious. Existentialism focuses on purpose and meaning in life, while religious concerns focus within a relationship, with God or Gods. The author agrees that the concept of spirituality is broader than religion and suggests that religion refers to the doctrine and practice within formal religious institutions.

Narayanasamy (1993) indicates that the spiritual dimension is broader than the institutionalised religion although its purposes can be incorporated within religious activities.

Elsdon (1995) considers the view that spiritual needs are distinct from religious needs and this creates an area of misunderstanding. She infers that everyone has spiritual needs, whether or not they are part of a formal religion; however, only some have religious needs.

Cornette (1997) defines spirituality as a dynamic within each human being – to situate one's self in a horizon that gives meaning to life's experience. Religion, she implies, is concerned with a particular form of spirituality that places the human being in relation to a god using elements such as a holy book, prayer, meditation or liturgy, or a group of like-minded people who out of their belief strive for a certain moral code.

Buber (1958) studied the human personality's religious and social dimensions. He links spirit with nature and the ongoing 'course of being' or existing.

Heidegger (1962) analyses time and being, and relates the spirit to actualisation in relation to time consciousness and self-consciousness.

Bailey (1997) acknowledges that a definition of religion is difficult, even within a theological context. He suggests that this is so as it underpins a deeper, more philosophical endeavour to define man, the soul and divinity. He cites Stanley Cook's (1918) understanding of the nature of life.

Hardy (1979) felt that unappeased religious desires could only be satisfied with spiritual philosophy. He commenced a systematic study of spiritual experiences. He acknowledged that the nature of spirituality is based on subjective feeling. He acknowledges the difficulty of identifying spiritual or religious philosophy in a world dominated by science. He suggests that a written record of subjective spiritual feelings and of the effects they have on the lives of people concerned would convince the intellectual world of their significance. His research has built up an academic knowledge to the understanding of the spiritual nature of man. He concluded from his study that the main characteristics of man's spirituality were transcendental reality, early childhood manifestations, a sense of presence, personalisation and prayer. He discussed the spiritual nature as meaning that which may not have a religious focus but that demonstrates a love of non-material things, such as natural beauty, music, art and moral values.

O'Connor (1988) suggests that more may be learnt about the patient's spiritual needs by questioning: 'What nourishes your spirit?' instead of 'What Church do you belong to?'. He urges professionals to be realistic and not assume that they will always have a positive effect. Some patients need to feel suffering and spiritual pain for specific reasons. He emphasises that changes occur and that continuous assessment is needed. He also highlights the fact that dying may raise spiritual issues but not necessarily spiritual pain. Spiritual care should not trigger inferences of faith healing or hocus pocus.

If staff are confused about their own spiritual awareness domain, then it is difficult for them to address patients' concerns. Millison & Dudley (1992) studied 117 professionals (49% nurses, 26% clergy, 14% social workers) and examined spirituality as an aspect of professional practice. While a great majority felt that spirituality played an important role in patient treatment, only 39% routinely initiated discussion about religion or spirituality during assessment. It was suggested that this could relate to the professional, ethical value of self-determination for the patient or the sensitivity inherent in spiritual issues. The study revealed that 18% reported that other staff, such as the pastoral counsellor, initiated discussion. The researcher suggested that other staff are subtly or overtly discouraged from exploring spiritual or religious material. All respondents used 'listening to patients talk about God' involving clergy or prayer. The researchers noted that meditation-guided imagery or dream interpretation was not used. This implied that most practitioners were more comfortable with 'God talk' rather than less-traditional approaches.

Wallace (1995) suggests that palliative care can be taught to any moderately competent clinician in 6 months or less: however, presence in the midst of despair of another and oneself cannot be taught. He deliberates as to whether the capacity to keep one's feet on the ground and heart open is a gift or a skill which one learns. He is cynical about the fact that so many hospices still exist, and that medicine still has not adopted the hospice philosophy as part of usual business within the practice of medicine.

Franco (1983) views death as a departure of spirit, or activating life principle, from material substances. He suggests that intervention may not necessarily be a specific creed prescribed by an organised religion, but that it may be a spiritual frame of reference viewed as a conscious denial of mortality. Franco admits to the ambiguity of the concept of spiritual support, indicating its interpretation may have an organisational religious slant or an individual's meaning to life and the present situation or a vague pastoral meaning.

Jung (1933) indicated that the spiritual problem of modern man relates to the fact that man is aware of the present. He sees the spirit as being within the body. Jung suggests that there is an attempt to transcend present levels of consciousness, which is modern man's way of dealing with the body and spirit in the here and now. He feels

a more hygienic approach to death would be to view it as a goal for which to strive; i.e. that shrinking away from death is abnormal and unhealthy and can rob the second half of life of its purpose.

Ballard et al (1999) identify that the need for cohesion and purpose in life is exacerbated in those facing terminal illness and death, and that God, or an existential other, can serve to blame or comfort, but nonetheless give purpose and meaning. Whichever tack the patient takes, care and support in such a spiritual dimension is an important part of health care, as pre- and post-operative management.

Theology has a bias towards belief systems and needs and spirituality is often viewed within a philosophical framework (Franco 1983). Hardy (1979) believed that unappeased religious desires could only be satisfied with spiritual philosophy. From his systematic study on people's spiritual experiences, he acknowledges that the nature of spirituality is based on subjective feelings which are influenced in a world dominated by science. Ballard (2000) suggests that spirituality could not automatically be equated with religion since, given the cultural history of our society, it tends to be restricted to Christianity in its highly institutionalised form.

THE USE OF TRANSITION MODELS TO RECOGNISE SPIRITUAL PAIN

Narayanasamy (1993) implies that chronic illness can bring about disorganisation and disruption, agreeing with Reed (1991) that patients suffering from chronic illness commonly experience intense spiritual awareness. Spiritual pain can then be viewed as existential distress as a consequence of the impact of disease and illness. Loveys (1990) suggests that a diagnosis of illness which can become chronic (such as advanced cancer), can be a time of profound personal crisis. She identifies the crisis as containing issues such as accepting diagnosis, informing a loved one and treatment and decision making. These issues relating to health and illness transition can result in spiritual pain in the transition period where there are crisis points. Murphy (1990) identifies issues including concept of loss, loss of identity, control and self-esteem, all of which can result in overwhelming existential distress or spiritual pain. The development of theoretical frameworks or models have enabled health professionals to conceptualise the process and offer intervention and support for patients who experience loss and spiritual distress as a result of a life-threatening illness. Bowlby (1986), Schneider (1984), Worden (1984) and Shlossberg (1981) all offer different theoretical perspectives. Bowlby focuses on the emotions and feelings relating to loss. Worden concentrates on tasks of mourning and Kubler Ross (1969) and Parkes (1971) discuss the stages of feelings like anger, denial, isolation and eventual acceptance. Sewart (1994) implies that the advantage of using a theoretical model for transition is that anticipation, and therefore intervention, by health professionals may enable some preparation for role change and possible avoidance of negative issues focusing on positiveness or hope. The role changes and transition experienced by Anne, a patient, are highlighted in relation to her spiritual pain in Case study 6.1.

Reimer & Davies (1991) emphasise the supportive role of nurses in enabling families' and patients' transitions between living with cancer and dying.

Hall (1997) suggests that there may be disadvantages in the use of models and theories relating to spiritual distress. She suggests that they can block intuition and routinise care, resulting in the loss of individual meaning. She compares professional knowledge and power in nurse/patient relationships, suggesting that it can disempower patients who, like Anne in the case study, are already experiencing loss of control as a result of transition. Pruen (1979) argues that the hospital environment can depersonalise patients. He suggests that fear of physical pain influences emotional

---

CASE STUDY 6.1

SPIRITUAL PAIN

History

Anne is a 48-year-old palliative care community nurse, happily married with a son of 24 years and a daughter aged 20. She was diagnosed with advanced ovarian cancer, and underwent pelvic surgery a week after diagnosis.

Surgery revealed a widespread cancer and she was advised that her prognosis was poor. She had aggressive chemotherapy and 6 weeks later suffered extensive hair loss accompanied by severe nausea. From there on her physical condition deteriorated rapidly. Within 6 weeks she had changed from a person with a role of health professional, wife and mother to a person in terminal decline.

She confided in a close relative that she was shocked, angry and frightened. She grieved that she would not live to see her children married, or future grandchildren born. She mourned the loss of a close and loving sexual relationship with her husband and she mourned the loss of status as a practising health professional.

Her role had changed from health professional to patient, from giver of care to recipient. She was now experiencing health care from a different perspective. It was, she said 'like being in a long, dark tunnel . . . no light . . . no breath . . . no spirit'.

Role change and transition

Anne was sustaining multiple losses and transitions, resulting in spiritual pain. Additionally, her illness and physical decline was untimely in the light of the life/death continuum. She experienced the transition from healthy professional, wife and mother, to becoming a patient unable to fulfil her role either as a professional or as a wife and mother. She also had to come to terms with the fact she was dying. She was experiencing spiritual pain.

Therapeutic dialogue from the visiting palliative care nurse enabled Anne to become almost objective about her situation. She focused on achieving realistic goals such as preparing for her daughter's 21st birthday party arrangements, which were imminent. This gave her a sense of meaning, purpose and hope. She said that the cycles in the garden, flowers opening and dying gave her a 'sense of reality and peace, of beginning and end'. This type of dialogue facilitated by the palliative care nurse helped her to become 'in touch with herself' in a way she had not been able to do with her family. She felt that this was because the almost bizarre topics would worry them and she 'wanted to wrap them in cotton wool and not give them more worry'.

Responses to questions

Question 1: Why is spirituality of interest to you?

The literature suggests that an open and broad question should be used as an icebreaker at the beginning of the session. This should enable all of the participants to contribute to the discussion (Kingry et al 1990). The initial findings were that, despite the moderators' offering an insight into what spirituality meant to them in understandable terms (Box 6.2), all of the males and 15 of the females found the concept of spirituality to be baffling. They focused mainly on religion, namely Christianity, which concurs with the majority of the literature (Narayanasamy 1993, Dyson et al 1997).

The researchers believe that this methodological approach allowed for appropriate personal disclosure, which appeared to encourage the participants to begin to reveal their thoughts and feelings, which could be an advantage when dealing with an emotive subject. Also, it could be argued that this method would not allow the participants to opt out by being in the 'security of the crowd' (Hansler & Cooper 1986) and, likewise, group safety could be seen to encourage the more reticent participant.

Question 2: What do you think people mean when they talk about spiritual things? Are they the same?

From the second question it became evident that the groups were beginning to focus their thoughts on aspects of spirituality other than religion and Christianity, but they did not continue to be a common feature. It also appeared that they were becoming challenging with their interactions and responses when comparing spirituality and religion. This probably occurred because they were already familiar with each other and bound by mutuality of their disease. Also, the moderators had prepared the groups by establishing ground rules, which included a statement explaining that there were no right or wrong answers and that they would be valued for their uniqueness. This was contradictory to the literature, which states that there may be forced compliance or a desire to be polite and fit within the norm.

Question 3: What are your spiritual needs? What would it be like if you did not have spiritual beliefs?

The groups responded differently: some were very clear on their needs and others were unsure, but on analysing the data it was apparent that common needs were identified, such as the need for inner peace; 'being with others who are in the same boat'; having meaning and purpose; empathy; belief/faith/prayer and hymns.

Even though it was felt that issues could have been clarified and explored at a deeper level during one-to-one interviews, the purpose of this study was to collate as much data as possible from the patient's perspective about these emotive issues. Also, a focus group interview is a data collection technique which capitalises on the interaction within a group to illicit rich experimental data (Asbury 1993), which was an invaluable approach for this exploratory study.

Question 4: How do you meet your spiritual needs? Who/what/support?

This particular question generated a range of responses regarding feelings, behaviours and attitudes relating to individual perception of spirituality. This supports the literature, which suggests that findings cannot be projected to the population at large (Hansler & Cooper 1986, Kruger 1994). So, it could be argued that a standard approach for spiritual care may not be appropriate, as there would be limited generalisability.

Question 5: Are there any things that you have particularly started to think about since your illness began?

The main themes that emerged related to mortality: feeling enforced and desired loneliness; moral values; increased awareness and appreciation of nature/art/music; bonding and development of friendships with those 'in the same boat'; and also being abandoned by friends who cannot cope with the cancer diagnosis.

Hansler & Cooper (1986) imply that findings cannot be automatically generalised to the population under question. This could be challenged in relation to this question as the researchers believe that, from their wealth of experience in this field, these would be the common issues raised for any individual facing a terminal illness. The researchers believe that one-to-one interviews could not necessarily identify common ground.

Question 6: How has your illness altered the way you see life?

The literature suggests that follow-up questions or probing is an important part of extracting full information from respondents. For example, there are some things that cannot be articulated easily, which is the case with this study, and probes may need to take the form of analogy (Sewart 1993, Kruger 1994).

This question generated the same answer as the previous one. It is believed that the second question built on the first, offering the participants an opportunity to think at a deeper level as both were very thought-provoking. It could be argued that the use of further probing would have gleaned richer information and, maybe, one-to-one interviews would have been appropriate with some participants.

Question 7: Have you become aware of something different around you since your illness began (communicating about spirituality)?

The main themes that were generated were the awareness of the time left and quality, valuing and sharing, being around people 'in the same boat', mutuality, avoidance tactics, overprotectiveness (both ways), vulnerability, more friends, abandoned, increased listening skills, empathy, calmness, past experiences, alienation, isolation and patience. It was clear from this question that this was not needed.

Question 8: Optional scenario

The literature states that a scenario may be useful to facilitate discussion. The researchers believe that the scenario was not effective with this group of individuals as they are often focusing on their illness and worries. Also, because of their rapidly changing disease process, it is difficult to be static enough to focus on an hypothetical situation. This may work well with a product evaluation in market research.

Question 9: Chaplaincy service: he/she should be male/female?

This question highlighted that numerous participants had damaging past experiences of religion. It was evident that these issues needed to be explored at a deeper level in a one-to-one interview.

The literature explored focused mainly on defining the term 'spirituality' and its ambiguity, which can result in vague and inappropriate approaches to spiritual care within the palliative care setting. The study explored the perception of palliative care patients regarding spirituality and how they would like to see this addressed. The methodological approach chosen was the use of focus groups, which elicited data from six groups (29 patients in total) within a regional palliative care centre. The literature suggests that larger numbers were needed than the groups in this study (four to six participants). However, the researchers believe that the results offered common and diverse data which can be used for further research.

Comparison was made with using one-to-one taped interviews. The results implied that the focus group approach was appropriate and valuable in discovering feelings and expectation about spirituality within a safe environment. During the group work only two individuals became upset, with both of them not wanting to opt out and seemingly comfortable with the group environment. Common themes emerged that suggests these patients regarded the bonding and being 'in the same boat' had enabled them to explore and share experiences about hope, life and indeed death. It was evident that the patients had a high regard for professionals, but it was clear that they did not feel that they would approach them to explore what they perceived to be spirituality. For practical purposes the approach enabled the data to be collected over a relatively short time.

Recommendations

- Focus groups can provide a safe environment, enabling patients to identify with others in the same boat, and express common feelings and emotions they may otherwise hide or feel are bizarre.
- The focus group approach can be used as an initial basis to explore issues such as patients' spiritual needs, which could then be followed by research exploring the perception of both carers and professionals.
- The results of this research project suggest that focus groups could be used as part of day centre or inpatient care, so that the spiritual needs of these patients may be addressed using a patient-centred approach.

CONCLUSION

The complexity of defining spiritual pain relates to the subjectivity of the individual's health/illness behaviour and where they are in life's continuum. The involvement, or not as the case may be, of life belief systems or religion can at times deflect the health professional's understanding and ability to identify and support patients experiencing spiritual pain during life-threatening illness. The use of a theoretical model or framework during transition experienced by patients with such conditions can assist practice, as far as the planning and intervention of care. The spiritual dimension of a person can be elusive to themselves and, therefore, sometimes difficult to recognise, let alone express. It is suggested that to enter the spiritual dimension of another, with a view to supporting and reducing spiritual pain, the health care professional should be able to

recognise their own spiritual dimension and address any defects. This may be facilitated by health care professionals using clinical supervision, and a more focused educational input relating to spirituality within all areas of health care, and in particular for those working with patients who have a life-threatening illness.

The study undertaken sought to throw light on the spiritual needs of patients, both through looking at a specific case study, and also in examining the role of focus groups as a supportive mechanism to enable patients to identify their own spirituality and spiritual needs. It is only through addressing and responding to the spiritual needs of patients that the health care professional and all those charged with care of patients can begin to fully deliver Cicely Saunders' philosophy of holistic care, which calls for consideration not only of the physical and psychological needs but also consideration of the spiritual needs of the patient.

The following check list could be used by those charged with the care of patients to ensure that those spiritual needs are addressed.

- Have I considered that the patient's pain may have a spiritual component?
- Have I made myself available for discussion?
- Have I made opportunities to discuss the meaning of the illness for the patient and family?
- Have I considered and discussed religious needs?
- Have I discussed the patient's care with a chaplain or spiritual adviser?
- Is the patient aware of religious services available?
- Have I allowed the patient time to discuss his/her thoughts as to the future?
- Have I, as a health care professional, a basic understanding of the differences between 'believers', agnostics, atheists, etc.?
- Do I understand what some people believe to be reincarnation?
- In the provision of physical care to the patient, have I taken into account the impact of that physical care on the patient's spirituality or beliefs: this may include the

role of diet, the role of personal hygiene, the personal needs for prayer, etc.

This list is not meant to be all-encompassing and, when considering other aspects of the holistic care of the patient, will need to be modified and amended to fully meet the individual needs of each patient.

ACKNOWLEDGEMENT

I would like to express my thanks to other members of the Research Team. The Research Team comprised: I. D. Finlay, P. Ballard, C. Searle, N. Owen and S. Roberts.

REFERENCES

Alderidge A D 1991 Spirituality, healing and medicine. British Journal of Medical Practice 41: 425–427

Asbury J E 1993 cited in Morgan D L (ed.) 1993 Successful focus groups – advancing the state of the art. Sage Publications, London

Atkinson J 1993 The patient as a sufferer. British Journal of Medical Psychology 6: 113–120

Bailey E 1997 Implicit religion in a contemporary society. KOK Pharos Pub. House, Germany

Ballard P 2000 Spiritual perspectives among terminally ill patients. A Welsh sample. Modern Believing 41(2): 30–38

Ballard P, Finlay I, Roberts S, Searle C, Jones H 1999 A perception of hospital chaplaincy. Contact 130: 27

Barnard D 1983 Religion and religious studies in healthcare education. Journal of Allied Health August: 192–200

Boutell K A, Bozett F W 1990 Nurses' assessment of spirituality: continuing education implications. The Journal of Continuing Education in Nursing 21(14): 172–176

Bowlby J 1986 Attachment and loss, sadness and depression. Basic Books, New York

Buber M 1958 I and thou, 2nd edn [translated by R G Smith]. T and T Clark, Edinburgh, pp. 159–161

Burnard P 1993 The spiritual needs of atheists and agnostics. The Professional Nurse Dec: 130–132

Cassell E 1982 The nature of suffering and the goals of medicine. The New England Journal of Medicine 306(11): 639–645

Cobb M 1997 Body and soul editorial. Progress in Palliative Care 5(4): 139–140

Cook S 1918 In: Hastings J (ed.) Religion in encyclopaedia of religions and ethics, Vol. X. T and T Clark, Edinburgh

Cornette K 1997 Forever I am weak, I am strong. International Journal of Palliative Nursing 3(1): 6–12

Domminian J 1983 The doctor as a prophet. British Medical Journal 287: 1925–1927

Dyson J, Cobb M, Forman D 1997 The meaning of spirituality: a literature review. Journal of Advanced Nursing 26: 1183–1188

Elsdon R 1995 Spiritual pain in dying people: the nurse's role. Professional Nurse 10(10): 641–643

Eshleman M 1992 Death with dignity: significance of religious beliefs and practices in hinduism, buddhism, and islam. Today's OR Nurse 14(11): 19–23

Franco V 1983 The hospice: humane care for the dying. Journal of Religion and Health 22(3): 241–249

Goddard N 1995 'Spirituality as integrative energy': a philosophical analysis as requisite precursor to holistic nursing practice. Journal of Advanced Nursing 22: 808–815

Grey A 1994 The spiritual component of palliative care. Palliative Medicine 8: 215–221

Hall B 1997 Spirituality in terminal illness: an alternative view of theory. Journal of Holistic Nursing 15(1): 82–96

Hansler D, Cooper C 1986 cited in Nyamathi A, Shuler P 1990 Focus Group interview: a research technique for informed nursing practice. Journal of Advanced Nursing 15: 1281–1288

Hardy A 1979 The spiritual nature of man, a study of contemporary religious experiences. Oxford University Press, Oxford

Heidegger M 1962 Being and time. Blackwell Publications, Oxford, p. 428

Jung C 1933 Modern man in search for his soul. Routledge, Keegan Paul, England

Kingry M J, Tiedje L B, Friedman L L 1990 Focus groups: a research technique for nursing. Nursing Research 39(2): 124–125

Kitzinger J 1995 Qualitative research – introducing focus groups. British Medical Journal 311: 299–302

Kruger R A 1994 Focus groups: a practical guide for applied research, 2nd edn. Sage, Thousand Oaks

Kubler Ross E 1969 On death and dying. Macmillan, London, pp. 14–15

Loveys B 1990 Transitions in chronic illness. The at risk role. Holistic Nursing Practice 4(3): 56–64

McGrath P 1999 Exploring spirituality through research: an important but challenging task. Progress in Palliative Care 7(1): 3–9

McKee D D, Chappel J N 1992 Spirituality and medical practice. The Journal of Family Practice 35(2): 201–208

McSherry W 1996 Raising the spirits. Nursing Times 92(3): 48–49

Martsolf D S, Mickley J R 1998 The concept of spirituality in nursing theories: differing world views and extend of focus. Journal of Advanced Nursing 27: 294–303

Mathers J 1976 In: Millard D W (ed.) 1976 Religion and medicine. Strategy and tactics of health care. SCM Press Ltd, London Institute of Religion, p. 83

Maughans T 1996 The spiritual history. Archives of Family Medicine 5: 11–16

Mickley J, Sochen Belcher A 1992 Spiritual well-being: religiousness and hope among women with breast cancer. Image: Journal of Nursing Scholarship 24(4): 267–272

Millard D W 1976 Towards a theology of social work. In: Millard D W (ed.) Religion and medicine. SCM Press Ltd, London Institute of Religion, p. 92

Millison M, Dudley J R 1992 Providing spiritual support: a job for all hospice professionals. The Hospice Journal 8(4): 49–65

Murphy S A 1990 Human responses to transitions. Holistic Nursing Practice 4(3): 1–7

Narayanasamy A 1993 Nurses' awareness and educational preparation in meeting their patients' spiritual needs. Nurse Education Today 13: 196–201

O'Connor P 1988 The role of spiritual care in hospice: are we meeting patients' needs? The American Journal of Hospice Care xx: 31–37

Parkes C M 1971 Bereavement studies of grief in adult life. Penguin, England

Pruen E 1979 The hospital: a place of truth. Nursing Times 15: 18

Reed P 1991 Preferences for spiritually related nursing interventions among terminally ill and non terminally ill hospitalised patients. Applied Nursing Research 4(3): 122–128

Reimer J C, Davies B 1991 Palliative care: the nurse's role in helping families through the transition of 'fading away'. Cancer Nursing 14(6): 321–327

Ross L 1994 Spiritual care – the nurse's role. Nursing Standard 8(29): 33–37

Saunders C 1988 Spiritual pain. Hospital chaplain. Bishop and Sons, Orpington, Kent

Schneider J 1984 Stress, loss and grief: understanding their origins and growth potential. University Pack Press, Baltimore, p. 61

Searle C, Finlay I, Owen J 1999 Spiritual needs: the role of focus groups to identify and address spiritual pain. Palliative Care Today VIII(iv): 52–54

Sewart D W 1993 Focus groups – theory and practice. Sage Publications, London, pp. 95–97

Sewart B M 1994 End of life decision making: from disclosure of HIV through bereavement. Scholarly Inquiry for Nursing Practice: An International Journal 8(4): 321–351

Shlossberg W 1981 A model for analysing human adaptation to transition. The Counselling Psychologist 9(2): 2–19

Spiritual Care Work Group 1990 Assumption and principles of spiritual care. Death Studies 14: 75–81

Turner P 1996 Caring more, doing less, palliative care. Nursing Times 92(34): 59–62

Wallace B 1995 Suffering, meaning and the goals of hospice care. The American Journal of Hospice and Palliative Care 12(3): 6–9

Watson J 1996 Art, caring, spirituality and humanity. In: Farmer E (ed.) Exploring the spiritual dimension of care. Quay Books, Mark Allen Publisher Ltd, Wiltshire

Worden W J 1984 Grief counselling and grief therapy. Springer, New York, p. 42

FURTHER READING

Amenta M 1988 Nurses as primary spiritual care workers. Hospice Journal 4(3): 47–55

Burnard P 1990 Learning to care for the spirit. Nursing Standard 4(18): 38–39

Carey M A 1993 cited in Morgan D L (ed.) 1993 Successful focus groups – advancing the state of the art. Sage Publications, London

Caterall R A, Greet B, Sankey J, Griffiths G 1998 The assessment and audit of spiritual care. International Journal of Palliative Nursing 4(4): 162–168

Cawley N 1997 An exploration of the concept of spirituality. International Journal of Palliative Nursing 3(1): 31–36

Dudley J, Smith C, Millison M 1995 Unfinished business: assessing the spiritual needs of hospice.... The American

Journal of Hospice and Palliative Care March/April: 30–37

Frankl V 1959 Man's search for meaning, 5th edn. Hodder and Stoughton, London

Hay M W 1989 Principles in building spiritual assessment tools. American Journal of Hospice Care 6(5): 25–31

Labun E 1988 Spiritual care an element in nursing planning. The Journal of Advanced Nursing 13: 314–320

National Council for Hospices and Specialist Care Services 1995 Specialist palliative care: a statement of definitions. Occasional paper 8, October

Renetzky L 1979 cited in Ross L 1994 Spiritual aspects of nursing. Journal of Advanced Nursing 19: 439–447

7

Complementary therapies

Sharon Macnish

INTRODUCTION

This chapter addresses some of the issues and concerns regarding the integration of complementary medicine in palliative care, with the emphasis on its use as an adjunct to nursing. I include a definition of complementary medicine and an overview of its popularity and advantages as well as its limitations. The philosophy and principles of complementary medicine are explored, many aspects of which are shared by palliative nursing. I propose that it is these similarities which have enabled palliative care nurses to utilise complementary medicine and integrate it into their body of skills. Some of the more popular therapies are discussed from nursing and patient perspectives and I address some of the professional issues raised.

Complementary medicine is a term used to describe many distinct therapies. Historically it describes anything that lies outside of established medical practice. It is a term which has referred to individual therapies as well as to traditional and complete systems of medicine which may have developed from other cultures.

For the purposes of this chapter I will use the following definitions:

• *Complementary medicine and complementary therapies* are terms used interchangeably. I will use both to describe therapeutic interventions designed to treat symptoms or minimise their effects. They may restore a sense of harmony and well-being to the individual. Although emphasis is placed upon an holistic approach, complementary medicine can be reductionist, in so far as the therapies do not pretend to be curative. The holistic approach is discussed later but includes a consideration of the patient's emotional, physical, mental, spiritual and creative needs when a treatment is chosen. Examples include aromatherapy, acupuncture, relaxation, massage and hypnotherapy.

- *Alternative medicine*: a complete system of medicine not taught by conventional medical training. It has clear diagnostic tools, investigations and treatment modalities purporting to treat the widest range of physical, psychological and mental illnesses. Thus it can stand apart from orthodox or conventional Western medicine. Examples include traditional Chinese medicine, Ayurvedic medicine, homeopathy and herbal medicine. Ethnic groups in Britain may be using these as mainstream medicine, including the treatment of cancer. Many alternative systems of medicine are only alternative to the West. They service the health care needs of significant sections of the world community where it is the Western system of medicine which is alternative (Bannerman et al 1983).

In Britain, conventional medicine is dominant and is used to treat cancer. Most people will seek an alternative treatment for cancer when conventional approaches have failed or the effects of treatment are considered detrimental. The more grim the prognosis and the more potentially damaging the proposed conventional intervention, the greater will be the tendency of patients to seek alternative sources of help. The role of alternative treatments for cancer is outside the remit of this chapter. Instead I will focus upon those therapeutic options which can be used as adjuncts to conventional palliative treatment and care.

THE UPTAKE OF COMPLEMENTARY MEDICINE

There are no 'facts in themselves', there are only facts for someone . . . for whom the fact is a fact.
(Pannikar, cited by Whitmont 1993 (p. 41))

The delivery of health care undergoes constant change in response to social, economic, political, educational and ethical considerations as well as developments in research. The growth in complementary and alternative medicine has occurred at a time when political and social changes have altered the relationship between the health care team and the patient. Issues concerning health can be viewed as part of a change in social consciousness. This includes new concepts such as:

- personal responsibility for actively feeling well
- a redefined relationship to nature
- the pursuit of preventative medicine.

Coward (1989, pp. 5–6) states that 'we are being encouraged to develop a much more loaded sense of health and well being' and that 'alternative therapies are both a spearhead and a symptom of widespread changes in attitude'. The Select Committee on Medical Ethics (1994) highlights the recent move away from paternalism and strongly endorses the right of the competent patient to refuse consent to any treatment. Modern ethical thinking advocates respect for autonomy and beneficence which results in the empowerment of patients (Gillon 1994). Other changes such as a more informed public and a positive media response to complementary medicine have contributed to a change in attitude. This has yet to be mirrored in real political change with regard to complementary and alternative medicine (Coward 1989).

Many people regard cancer and other life-threatening diseases as random events to which one attempts to bring meaning. Illness is, however, not a rational event but an experiential one. Unfortunately, too often, the available treatments seldom take account of the subjective inner world of the patient. Instead they focus on objective elements which are regarded in many medical models to be the whole of illness.

It is generally accepted that illness disrupts us in different ways and may be affected by the stage and severity of disease as well as the age and development of the individual experiencing the event. It may attack our sense of integrity and wholeness. The accompanying changes to self-worth and self-concept may be expressed at the physical, cognitive, behavioural, emotional, spiritual, interpersonal and sexual levels. Short-term physical, psychological and spiritual help is often required as people gradually adapt to the abnormal situation that accompanies a frightening diagnosis. Addressing this problem is a fundamental requirement of nursing. Interestingly, it is nurses who have most readily responded to public demand for complementary types of treatment and applied them in practice, particularly in palliative care (Rankin-Box 1997). My contention is that the philosophical basis of nursing, complementary medicine and palliative care are similar and that it is in nursing that the most fruitful connections may occur to provide benefit to the patient. This is explored later in the chapter.

OVERVIEW OF ORTHODOX AND COMPLEMENTARY MEDICINE

The pertinent question is not how to do things right but how to find the right thing to do, and to concentrate resources and effort on them.
(Peter F. Drucker)

In Britain, which provides free treatment at the point of delivery of care, it may seem extraordinary that people are willing to pay for additional and different health care. This may reflect a greater degree of information and choice about health, but it could reflect dissatisfaction or unease with aspects of conventional treatment, as well as failures in self-medication.

All systems of medicine are partial and, therefore, limited. Medicine has evolved from the philosophical and religious traditions of unique and particular cultures. Porter (1997, p. 7), explains that 'most traditional healing systems have sought to understand the relations of the sick person to the wider cosmos and to make readjustments between individuals and the world, or society and the world, the western medical tradition explains sickness principally in terms of the body itself – its own cosmos'. This partiality is reflected worldwide. The traditional Chinese system of medicine reflects a Chinese philosophical and social view of what constitutes a human being. It differs from the system of medicine used by Native Americans, which reflects their values and beliefs. Likewise, the European and American systems of medicine reflect the various traditions, values and beliefs of each culture. This results in significant differences in the ways that the same disease is treated in each country. These differences occur not as a result of research and differing resources but as a direct reflection of the beliefs and values about illness and cure as expressed by that culture (Payer 1990).

Europe and America have some philosophical commonality in the shared view which has dominated Western thought since the time of Descartes (1596–1650). He conceived of the philosophical concept that separated attributes of the mind, such as logic and conceptual thinking, from other less rational and subjective mental functions, such as feelings and intuition. This was an intellectual concept which ensured that nothing was held to be true until there were established grounds for believing it to be true. One result was that in medicine, the study of the body, its function and the effect of disease upon it became the dominant focus. Aspects of mental and spiritual function, such as consciousness, creativity, emotions, beliefs, subjectivity, thoughts, feelings and experience, were largely excluded from study. For centuries the notion of the mind and spirit as causative factors in illness and health was subjugated to the study of the body, or ignored altogether in the West. These psychological, emotional and spiritual links are only now being investigated with a degree of rigour (Pelletier 1977, Moyers 1993). It is important to realise that this spiritual/mental/physical split did not occur in cultures very different from our own. Their aims, objectives and treatments may appear unusual compared to ours. The reason is that the philosophical concepts underpinning other systems of medicine could not permit treatment of the body alone.

Generally the practice of orthodox Western medicine continues to pursue reductionism, which has contributed enormous advances in the understanding of disease. A critical examination of the relationship between the mind and the body is a recent phenomenon in Western science, although the relationship has been acknowledged as powerful since time immemorial. Indeed, the ongoing attempts to separate body and mind remain a central tenet in clinical trials of drugs where a placebo response is anticipated and accounted for in a trial protocol, thus maintaining the delusion that the universe and its component parts are predictable. This is not to negate the strengths of the biomedical model, which forms one useful tool that can be used to test a hypothesis. Holistic approaches to research accept that subjectivity directly influences the observable physical world and is unpredictable. Living systems function as wholes, each whole profoundly affecting and being affected by another. This permits research into phenomena such as self-healing and spontaneous remission as well as opening up the possibilities of investigation into unconventional treatments.

Recent research in psychoneuroimmunology, which examines links between the mind, the immune system and the nervous system, reveals that the interrelationship between them is much more complex than expected at the molecular level (Pert 1997). While this means that it is no longer in question that the mind and emotions have an effect upon the immune and nervous systems, the overall impact they have upon disease and any promise of cure this offers remains impossible to correlate. The subtle levels of healing as examined by writers such as Gerber (1988) and Talbot (1991), and which form the basis of belief and practice in many cultures, has as yet, hardly been researched.

Medicine continues to make advances in surgery, diagnostic techniques and complex treatment regimens, ensuring that the knowledge base increases exponentially. This places fresh demands upon health care professionals to achieve higher standards of training, competence and specialisation. Subsequently, there is less time spent in developing the human-centred skills of communication and empathy which form important elements of a good therapeutic relationship. Authors such as Buckman & Sabbagh (1994) claim that complementary practitioners have the time and attention to develop good communication skills which enhance the therapeutic value of a consultation. They purport

that this, and the placebo effect, account for most of the apparent success of complementary medicine. However, Kienle & Kiene (1998) have analysed the published literature on placebo and conclude that there is insufficient evidence for the existence of any therapeutic placebo effect. Nevertheless, conventional treatment continues to treat disease rather the individual and many question the effect that some drugs and interventions have upon long-term health and vitality. Therapies such as osteopathy, homeopathy, massage, healing and acupuncture, once viewed with hostility and suspicion, are now being reconsidered. Perhaps they are perceived as being gentler, effective, less-invasive and more supportive to the individual who is seeking help, often short term, at many levels. This is particularly relevant for any chronic, long-term disease where the prospect for cure is poor.

In summary:

- The delivery of health care is not static and responds dynamically to change.
- Cancer and other chronic conditions are experiential events and require a range of therapeutic options which acknowledge this reality and support patients through their experience.
- The biomedical paradigm has no framework to include this human experience, therefore treatments address the physiological mechanisms alone.
- Holistic paradigms reinstate subjectivity and consciousness into scientific debate and research.
- Complementary medicine offers therapeutic options to support a patient experiencing life-challenging events. Research into the effectiveness of complementary medicine can be achieved through biomedical *and* holistic methodologies, including quantitative and qualitative methods.

THE PHILOSOPHY OF COMPLEMENTARY MEDICINE

Soul is not a thing, but a quality or a dimension of experiencing life and ourselves. It has to do with depth, value, relatedness, heart and personal substance.   (Thomas Moore 1992, p. 5)

Complementary medicine differs from conventional medicine in its philosophy, principles and in some of the practices and methods it uses.

Some systems of medicine have clear diagnostic techniques and are genuinely alternative. They may originate entirely from another culture, such as traditional Chinese medicine, and will, therefore, reflect that culture rather than our own. Nevertheless, there has been a rich plundering of techniques from alternative systems of medicine which Westerners have separated from their philosophical base and used for symptom control, sometimes with excellent results. The following example demonstrates this and emphasises the difference between the biomedical and holistic paradigms: in Britain, Western-trained doctors and nurses who use acupuncture frequently apply it for pain control based on the evidence of endorphin release at determined needle insertion points. They make no reference to the diagnostic tools of pulse and tongue diagnosis used in traditional Chinese medicine because there is no shared philosophical view of ourselves as *energetic* entities interacting with the cosmos. Our belief system may make it impossible to accept the conceptual and energetic measurements of Yin, Yang and elemental patterns which are considered of primary importance by Eastern practitioners. Oriental doctors would seldom apply acupuncture alone because it is considered too strong, particularly for debilitated patients. Acupuncture might be applied after an energetic diagnosis, and it would precede dietary and lifestyle changes plus herbal treatments. These would be used first to correct biochemical imbalance and restore strength, vitality and harmony at more than the physical level.

Some of the vital philosophical differences between alternative medicine, complementary medicine and orthodox medicine are a result of the separation of body, mind, spirit (or vibration) and environment in diagnosis and treatment. Indeed, this can be expanded in that holistic practitioners of alternative and complementary medicine consider that there are five layers or components to being whole: spirit, mind, emotion, vitality and the biochemical body.

Vitality is the concept that life is a dynamic force; i.e. life is an energetic process directed from within. Each individual is considered to have a purposeful internal energy that actively seeks to be healthy. Symptoms are thus viewed differently, and are not necessarily undesirable. They may not always represent pathology and, instead, provide an indication that body–mind is attempting to maintain equilibrium in the face of disturbance. Some practitioners such as Vithoulkas (1980) regard the suppression of troubling symptoms as unwise, because some symptoms may be the successful attempt of the organism to achieve homeostasis. To suppress symptoms is to risk driving them deeper into the body or psyche. Remaining mindful of any developing pathology, treatment is designed to mitigate the pain and suffering caused by symptoms, while at the same time eliminating cause. Treatment is always intended to encourage the body's innate ability to correct defects or at least adapt to them within well-defined parameters. This is of course precisely the aim of palliative care.

An aspect of vitality that is seldom addressed is the importance of the environment. Western medicine has relied upon pharmacology for the development of drugs and has paid scant attention to cures from plants. This has placed it at odds with the environment, a situation that is slowly being recognised. By contrast, many traditional systems of medicine have a cosmological view that supports the environment (Arvigo 1995). Thus, the abuse and destruction of the habitat is unthinkable, not least because it feeds us and provides medicine. Food as medicine, diet as therapy and programmes of fasting and cleansing often form major treatments in traditional and alternative forms of medicine. Vitality in food is not about vitamins and minerals but is concerned with the life force of the plant and how it is grown and consumed. Coward (1989) argues against the romantic and sentimental view of nature used to promote alternative and complementary medicine. She notes that on the whole political change has not occurred as a result of changes in social consciousness and ecology, which is so closely reflected in the alternative health movement. In traditional societies which depend on plants and herbs for medicine, topics such as ecology, the interaction with nature, land rights and management issues are neither romantic nor sentimental but are the essence of their survival.

Because many of these philosophical differences affect practice, I believe that they must be considered if there is to be a successful integration of the therapies into palliative care. An example would be the use of concentrated plant essences used in aromatherapy. In the process of plant distillation, pollutants concentrate in the beneficial essential oils and it can be argued that only organic essential oils, taken from sustainable and replenishable sources, should be used in holistic health care. As with all aspects of medicine and nursing, ethical considerations have a cost attached. Complementary medicine has no advantage of truth and there are no right or wrong answers for how it can be applied:

- All too frequently complementary medicine is viewed as an adjunct for symptom control. Time-consuming holistic assessment and treatment modalities are ignored.
- Fortunately the philosophy of palliative care and holistic nursing share many of the values of complementary medicine, including the emphasis on the therapeutic relationship. These values are discussed later.

COMPLEMENTARY MEDICINE IN PALLIATIVE CARE

> He thought he saw an Argument
> That proved he was the Pope:
> He looked again, and found it was
> A Bar of Mottled Soap.
> 'A fact so dread,' he faintly said.
> 'Extinguishes all hope'.
> (Lewis Carroll)

While an examination of the wide range of therapeutic applications is outside the scope of this chapter, it is useful to consider several therapies which are most popularly used by nurses in palliative care (Rankin-Box 1997). These are the physical therapies concerned with touch and the senses as well as the mental therapies concerned with emotions and empowerment.

Relaxation and guided imagery

The physiological mechanisms which connect mind and body lie at the heart of relaxation and guided imagery. A central belief is that what a person believes, thinks and feels affects every cell in the body. Imagery (thoughts, pictures, sounds, memories, feelings, sensations) forms the basis of how we experience ourselves – our bodies, our relationships, our work, our environment and our emotional and spiritual lives. Guided imagery makes conscious and creative use of this faculty, to create a psycho–physiological change to reduce stress, adjust to change, and promote health and healing. Patients develop ways of tapping into the powerful resources of the mind to affect physical, psychological or spiritual change according to their needs. Practice may increase the capacity to change limiting beliefs, thoughts and feelings, to enhance relaxation and promote healing. In my experience, many patients quickly respond to this, enjoying the fact that they have some control over events in their life and the part that they are able to contribute to the healing process. As with any other therapeutic intervention, there are pitfalls, dangers and contraindications for the use of guided imagery. A common concern arises because patients have been left with a sense of guilt for having caused their cancer (or failed to cure it) because of perceived faults and psychological or spiritual blocks in their lives. Guilt and remorse are ordinary human emotions which can be sympathetically addressed without re-enforcement. This is expressed by Moore (1992), who argues for the reintegration of science and art in healing. He states that:

a poetic reading of the body as it expresses itself in illness calls for a new interpretation for the laws of imagination. . . . In recent years some have spoken against a metaphoric view of disease because they don't want us blaming patients for their physical problems. . . . Rather than blame, we should respond. Listening to the messages of the body is not the same as blaming patients.   (Moore 1992, p. 159)

Many patients will actively seek to understand and resolve their emotional and spiritual pain using techniques such as counselling, relaxation and guided imagery. The issue for nurses is how best to offer advice or how to train in these therapies and avoid the simplistic 'solutions' of popular self-help books and courses. These risk leaving patients unsupported when they are most vulnerable.

Massage and other touch-based therapies

For many the need for touch is as vital in illness as it is in health and yet it is poorly researched in nursing and in palliative care, perhaps because touch is an ill-defined concept (Estabrooks & Morse 1992). Researchers investigating the use of touch in nursing generally describe it within two categories. The first category is touch incidental to nursing activities, such as wound dressing, bathing and manual handling. Practically based, it is task-oriented and attends to the patient's physical needs. It frequently has a caring component in its delivery. The second category is variously described as expressive (McCann & McKenna 1993) or caring (Estabrooks 1989). It describes touch which conveys empathy, caring and concern and it is more emotionally motivated. Both forms of touch can be fraught with difficulties both for nurse and patient. These include misinterpretation of intent and meaning across culture and gender; inappropriate response to a personal and private situation; and violation of personal space. Macnish (1998) highlights the challenges faced by community palliative care nurses who work in isolation and concludes that 'little evidence currently exists to guide nurses into the best way of delivering appropriate, effective and helpful touch in practice'. Perhaps therapists and nurses who have trained in massage are more comfortable with touching, because their training provides the structure and boundaries to avoid many of the pitfalls inherent in expressive touch. If consent is given for a foot massage with a clearly defined aim such as relaxation, then there is a reduced possibility for misinterpretation by patients, family and colleagues.

A variety of touch-based techniques are utilised for symptom control, stress management and for the restoration of positive body image. Examples include acupressure for the relief of nausea, acupuncture for pain control and massage for insomnia. Touch therapies have a useful role to play in helping to restore the sense of sensuality, physical attractiveness and sexuality which is generally so poorly addressed in nursing (Gamlin 1999). I have often felt humbled by the responses to some of the simple and time-limited massages I have given, such as a foot massage. Some of the most moving and emotional responses have been from the elderly who have possibly not been touched for many years. Their sense of joy and gratitude in receiving tender, respectful, appropriate and loving touch has reminded me that we remain sensual and sexual beings until we die. Others have responded with outpourings of grief as the part of their body most ravaged by surgery and radiotherapy has been touched. Opportunities are created for talking and the sharing of experiences, both painful and joyful. This may be as important and relevant for the patient as other aspects of their care which are met through orthodox practices. Concerns about the spread of cancer by massage are unsubstantiated by research and a study by McNamara (1994) addresses many points raised by this.

Aromatherapy

The use of essential plant oils to combat disease and relieve symptoms is well established in France (Franchomme 1980) and other European countries but is poorly utilised here. In Britain, aromatherapy was introduced by the beauty industry and was later incorporated for stress management combined with massage. Although many therapeutic uses for essential oils are recognised, the stress reduction properties of the oils is most powerfully advocated in palliative care. Nurses have introduced the oils into their clinical environment, either through the fragrance route or through topical application via inhalation, baths or massage. Some disquiet has been expressed about the introduction of essential oils in this way, as very little evidence has been compiled for their efficacy or otherwise in clinical practice. Several recent textbooks by Buckle (1997), Price & Price (1995) and Tisserand & Balacs (1995) have attempted to address some of the safety, legal and professional issues involved in the practice of aromatherapy. Nevertheless, this author's experience supports the evidence emerging from reviews by the NHS Confederation (1997) and the Foundation for Integrated Medicine (1997) that many nurses are using aromatherapy without adequate training, safety protocols, management guidelines and indemnity insurance. Professional issues are examined later in this chapter.

Advantages of complementary medicine for the patient

- Many of the therapies provide an opportunity to learn new skills which can help a person gain control. Such skills may reduce the sense of helplessness which frequently accompanies a cancer diagnosis, e.g. guided imagery for pain control.
- Many of the therapies require the active participation of the patient, who is expected to work toward recovery or improvement and to achieve something for her or himself. The power base is shifted toward the patient, who is usually kept fairly passive and disempowered by the technological interventions of conventional medicine.
- The time such intervention takes is greater than a conventional one. This allows the sharing and exchange of information and provides an opportunity for patients to be heard and recount their own unique stories.
- Complementary medicine offers non-pharmacological options for symptom control and reduces the drug risk for patients; e.g. acupuncture for pain, relaxation for anxiety, aromatherapy for sleeplessness.
- Complementary medicine may provide physical contact and intimacy, e.g. therapeutic massage from a therapist or family. Touch therapies provide an opportunity to return to the innate skill of meaningful touch which has its own non-verbal language and allows the body to speak and communicate.

- Complementary medicine can reconnect the individual to her/his emotional and spiritual self.
- Complementary medicine frequently augments and strengthens the effects of other treatments.
- The patient often experiences immediate results, although these may be short term.

It is important to view these benefits with objectivity and to consider some possible disadvantages of using complementary medicine.

Disadvantages of complementary medicine for the patient

- There is no such thing as a completely safe therapy. Any intervention has potential hazards and this must be examined by all parties involved.
- Some people prefer passivity in their treatment and will not welcome decision making, empowerment and change when they are just about coping.
- Without adequate funding for complementary medicine, it remains too expensive for the majority to afford. This keeps valuable treatment options available to middle-income earners and is inequitable.
- Each doctor and nurse has a duty of care and is, therefore, vicariously liable for any referral made to a complementary practitioner. Most doctors know very little about complementary medicine (NHS Confederation 1997). Subsequently, they remain reluctant to make a professional referral without a greater depth of knowledge of the therapy concerned and a reasonable level of confidence in the therapist.

While arguments continue about safety, efficacy and funding for complementary medicine the patient perspective is often the one to which least attention is paid.

Case study 7.1, which emphasises more clearly the benefits that can be experienced by an integrated approach to cancer treatment and palliative care, features a woman who was aged 44 when she was diagnosed with breast cancer, and tells of her experiences in her own words.

CASE STUDY 7.1

USE OF INTEGRATED APPROACH FOR CANCER TREATMENT AND PALLIATIVE CARE

I was diagnosed with breast cancer in April 1994. No matter who you are, no matter what the circumstances, any life-threatening diagnosis sends the most violent shock waves through the body. The night of the diagnosis, my body took over totally and started to shake uncontrollably. My temperature dropped to what felt like minus zero! I was quite simply terrified and in a state of shock. In May I underwent that almost symphonic sounding procedure 'lump and lymph'. The tumour and several lymph nodes were removed and I was sent home 2 days later with a drain under my arm, feeling quite unreal.

I still needed to be in control and to make it OK for everyone around me, but I was beginning to feel the stirring of something that was not OK and that was in need of caring. I believe now that this was the soul.

Already, my body was taking the brunt of my psychological processes, which insisted I kept control. I was not allowing the body to be just where it was – shocked, bruised and hurting. The dearest of friends who had stayed with me in hospital and who was with me then, lit a candle, and as we talked she gently asked how I felt about having some body treatment such as aromatherapy. It was the most loving and supportive of suggestions from someone who knew better than anyone of my deep fear of body work and what a forbidden area it was for me. My reaction surprised me. I knew that massage with essential oils was frowned upon by some doctors and I had never dared to have any body treatment up until then. But, I experienced a huge wave of longing when I was asked this question and I said yes to it. This was a time when I heard my soul speak.

The person recommended to me was a trained nurse as well as a clinical aromatherapist, which helped enormously. And so, a few days after commencing chemotherapy, clinical aromatherapy entered my life. A gentle start, just hands and feet, but it was enough to establish trust and a rapport. I was amused that the parts of my body not touched objected to being left out! I received chemotherapy every third week for 8 months. The nurses were kind, gentle and extremely skilled but even so it was the most invasive, pervasive and horribly debilitating treatment. To then receive, not just the benefits of the essential oils themselves, but also such gentle, loving and healing touch was, I believe, as life-saving as any medical intervention and it was certainly more life enhancing! Perhaps more so because it went beyond the realms of the body and helped to reach and heal my mind, my heart and my soul.

The massage proceeded to arms, shoulders and legs, and I was able to receive help for my affected arm, horribly swollen, numb and yet painful, which had resulted from my surgery. I was learning to communicate with my aromatherapist and ask for help when things were not OK. A great deal of trust is needed to have any sort of treatment, be it allopathic, complementary, alternative or whatever. To have someone qualified as a nurse with experience of dealing with the very sick was important. To have someone with clinical knowledge of oils is in my experience, essential. My tumour was oestrogen-receptive, and so it is advisable that oils do not stimulate the body's production of oestrogen. The nausea caused by the chemotherapy is created at two sources: the chemoreceptor trigger zone in the brain and in the stomach. Oils can be balanced to support both areas, as indeed are the anti-nausea drugs prescribed. Once my body adjusted to the oils I was able to greatly reduce the dose of oral antiemetics and thus eliminate some medication. After chemotherapy, I commenced daily radiotherapy for 7 weeks. Some people burn more than others and I listened to my soul again when accepting a very specific blend of oils to soothe a very burnt and sore nipple and areola. Again my 'good girl' tapes were quieted by this still calm voice of the soul.

Many people are able to accept body work as a matter of course and that's wonderful. I would simply emphasise that for all, this is a time when it is more essential than ever before. But for each individual, it is first and foremost essential to be able to have the time and space to listen to their own hearts, to listen to that soul voice that does speak to us all.

My first nurse left the UK and referred me to a colleague and, although I was apprehensive about the change, it worked wonderfully well. This therapist was also a herbalist. When I started heavy and persistent uterine bleeding for 8 months, attributed to tamoxifen, I was given help with herbs and advice on sustaining my general health as so much blood loss was taking its toll. Throughout all this, I also received spiritual healing from a dear and trusted friend, which I am sure has contributed to my healing and recovery.

There has been another vital element for me in this approach to health care. Both aromatherapists were very firm with me and both had a lovely sense of humour – an essential ingredient to carry on in the grim times. The humour never belittled nor ignored the severity of what I was experiencing, but it kept it all in balance and kept me in touch with the light and the fact I was more than the cancer. Neither nurse ever treated me as a 'cancer patient'. They didn't treat the cancer, they treated the whole of me.

I have the greatest respect for the medical and nursing teams who were responsible for my care and may be again. But they only have that responsibility if I give it to them. Ultimately everything is my responsibility. I had to make many major decisions after hearing many differing opinions. Even when there was no agreement between medical teams about the best options for me, and a decision seemed impossible for me to make, I accepted that the ultimate responsibility and choice was mine. When this happens there is

only one court of appeal, the soul. I believe that we all have so much healing capacity within ourselves but that we must take the time to be still and listen to what our whole needs are in body, mind, feelings and soul. I never envisaged a situation in my life where soul would speak so loudly. Looking back now, my only regret is that I did not have aromatherapy and healing from the moment of diagnosis.

HOLISTIC NURSING IN PALLIATIVE CARE; THE WAY FORWARD FOR THE INTEGRATION OF COMPLEMENTARY MEDICINE?

And slow things are beautiful;
  The closing of day,
The pause of the wave
  That curves downward to spray,
The ember that crumbles,
  The opening flower,
And the ox that moves on
  In the quiet of power.
(Elizabeth Coatsworth)

In Britain, nurses have recently seen their role change. There have been changes in education and management plus extensive changes in NHS structure which are examined elsewhere in this book. Nursing is being critically appraised and many assumptions are being challenged. Many argue that nursing is undergoing a paradigm shift and that radical change is required if nursing is to develop meaningfully (Wright 1995). Technology fragments nursing and dominates it at the expense of caring and of collective and individual values, all of which are necessary if healing is to occur. Nursing must embrace the qualitative side of health care and the therapeutic role. This requires a re-examination of our role in healing as well as our social perceptions about the meaning of illness in order that nursing fulfils the public expectation that its practitioners provide the human face of the health care system.

Holistic nursing is not new, but traditional hierarchical nurse roles do not promote or encourage such an approach. Self-awareness lies at the heart of holistic nursing. Without the opportunity to explore this and develop skills as part of nursing education programmes, it is

unreasonable to expect inexperienced nurses to learn from their seniors who have not been exposed to such skills themselves. New models of nursing attempt to address this by introducing holistic concepts and they try to provide a framework for integration into practice. An example is Davies & Oberle's (1990) model of palliative nursing shown in Figure 7.1. The overall dimension of valuing has global and personal implications and holds within it five other interwoven dimensions. These are connecting; doing for; finding meaning; empowering; and preserving own integrity. In this example, preserving own integrity provides the emphasis missing from traditional models which still dominate practice. Exploring our emotions, and subjective inner experiences as nurses helps us to develop appropriate coping strategies as we look inward. Self-care is implicit, as is personal development, not only in terms of knowledge and skills but also of the psyche and the soul. Permitting self-examination of established attitudes and nursing practices contributes to the behavioural changes necessary if nursing is to demonstrate an intrinsically therapeutic role. I believe that nursing, in its wholeness, is therapeutic. However, I need to be able to demonstrate that who I am as a nurse combined with what I do as a nurse, reduces suffering, supports healing and promotes the education and well-being of my patients. Without this, task allocation and the division of patient care remains an economic and politically expedient way to reduce budgets within the continuing constraints of the health service.

Perhaps in the process of providing complementary therapies to patients, nurses are providing something precious for themselves: they

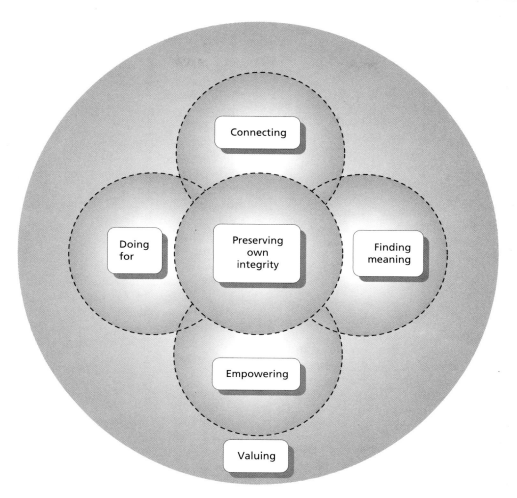

Figure 7.1   Dimensions of the nurse's supporting role, from Davies B & Oberle K (1990) with kind permission of Oncology Nursing Press.

are reclaiming an aspect of nursing which they perceive is no longer valued either by training and assessment procedures, or by purchasers of health care and managers. These are values which are concerned with healing, love, caring and compassion (Wright 1995). The training in, and practice of, complementary medicine may enhance intuitive and creative skills which can balance the high technological skills also required of nurses. The use of complementary medicine is not, however, different from other skills used by nurses. It is holistic practice which redefines nursing, not complementary medicine.

Some of the shared concepts and values of complementary medicine, holistic nursing and palliative care can be summarised as follows:

• All have a philosophy which is concerned with holism and holistic practice. Body, mind and spirit are all connected and have everything to do with health and well-being.
• Each of the therapies emphasises a person's uniqueness and attempts to tailor treatment to meet varied and changing needs. This includes understanding and treating people in the context of their culture, their family and their community.

- Each of the therapies includes the use of therapeutic approaches that mobilise an individual's unique and innate capacity for self-healing at many levels and that support living and dying well.
- Holistic practice is based upon equal participation and partnership. There is a greater emphasis on helping people to understand and help themselves, on education and on self-care rather than dependence. This involves entering into a non-dependent relationship with the patient, and places demands upon its practitioners for maintaining boundaries and changing behaviour so that each stays well. Holistic practice transforms the practitioners as well as the patient.
- Illness can be viewed as a possible opportunity for discovery as well as misfortune if a person so chooses. The dying process is an essential journey for the soul, which embraces each person's spiritual belief.
- Holistic practice includes an understanding of the social and economic conditions that generate and maintain ill health. A commitment to challenge this includes efforts to improve the therapeutic value of the environment in which health care takes place.

Bringing benefit to clients is integral to holistic practice. As the evidence of efficacy and benefit of complementary medicine and the therapeutic relationship increases, so nursing develops in therapeutic value.

PROFESSIONAL ISSUES

Several reports on the use of complementary medicine in the NHS indicate that it remains a marginal activity (Foundation for Integrated Medicine 1997, NHS Confederation 1997). Both of these reports identify key factors which must be resolved so that the uptake of complementary medicine evident in the private sector can be met by the NHS. While neither document specifically addresses palliative care, it is likely that similar reservations inhibit the uptake of complementary medicine by the organisations which deliver it in hospices and the community.

Safety and efficacy

Alternative and complementary medicine is emerging at a time when orthodox health care and practice is being scrutinised for evidence of both safety and efficacy. Many accepted medical, surgical and nursing practices have evolved without this scrutiny and will require review. Eddy (1994) points out that only 15% of medical interventions are supported by solid scientific evidence, partly because medical treatments are largely unassessed and partly because only 1% are scientifically sound. If this is the case, with the vast resources and research skills available to conventional medicine, it is relevant in any demand for rigorous scientific research in complementary medicine, notoriously underfunded by research bodies and the pharmacological industry. It is unlikely that evidence will become available in the short term to accelerate the integration of complementary medicine within the NHS. This is recognised by the Foundation for Integrated Medicine (1997), which urges government funding to conduct large-scale trials. In the meantime, nurses using complementary medicine should be practising within agreed protocols with written standards to ensure safety. Furthermore, with good evaluation tools and audit, results could be shared through organisations such as the Royal College of Nursing Forum on Complementary Medicine. These measures would promote the early stages of evidence-based practice in nursing.

Training and competency

Most complementary therapy training in Great Britain does not meet an agreed standard and is variable. Many complementary medicine organisations are attempting to rationalise training standards and offer continuing education as well as codes of practice and disciplinary procedures. The Osteopaths Act 1993 and Chiropractors Act 1994 now regulate these professions. It is likely that acupuncture, homeopathy and herbal medicine will seek similar protected status over the next decade. Self-regulation is most likely for the remaining smaller professional bodies which represent many complementary therapies. In the meantime most training courses in complementary medicine have not been designed with the nurse in mind. This may change slowly as training in complementary medicine is offered by universities who specifically target health care professionals and who link that education to an appropriate regulatory organisation. Because nurses work in such a variety of complex environments and are governed by professional codes of conduct, they have additional responsibilities when using complementary medicine as an adjunct to their nursing skills. Each nurse has a professional responsibility to ensure that the level of training is adequate for practice in palliative care and that the practice is safe and in the patient's best interest. Training must be of a sufficient depth and duration to allow for both supervised practice and reflection.

Lack of knowledge of a therapy

There is little if any familiarisation with complementary or alternative medicine in medical and nursing schools (British Medical Association 1993, Foundation for Integrated Medicine 1997). This could be resolved if undergraduate training included a common component which explored complementary medicine. This could be balanced in the private sector if its training schedules in complementary medicine included a more rigorous examination of orthodox science and clinical medicine in the syllabus (Foundation for Integrated Medicine 1997).

When presenting a proposal to integrate a therapy into clinical practice it must have clear aims which acknowledge the limitations as well as the benefits of any proposed therapy. Gaining team support is essential. I believe that experiential learning remains the most powerful method of helping team members appreciate the benefits of the complementary approach. By offering and encouraging the uptake of a staff service, health care professionals can experience them for themselves. At the same time it provides managers with the opportunity to demonstrate

the value that they place on their staff. It may even help to alleviate the stresses that carers experience in the provision of a palliative care service.

In summary:

• Funding, resources and research personnel for complementary medicine are lacking.
• Most trials for safety and efficacy of a product or procedure are funded by the pharmacological industry or orthodox and well-funded charities: neither shows great interest in supporting complementary medical research.
• Large-scale research into complementary medicine requires government funding.
• Nurses using complementary medicine must work within agreed protocols and standards of practice. This should include well-designed evaluation tools and audit in order to promote evidence-based practice. Pilot studies could form an essential part of this evidence.
• No single intervention is intrinsically safe and safety issues must take priority prior to planning.
• Each nurse has a legal obligation to demonstrate competence for the use of complementary medicine in a specific situation.
• Reflection on practice, good communication and clear documentation promote the use of complementary medicine.
• Gaining team support for complementary medicine is essential. Aim for resolution and understanding, not conflict.
• Experiential learning introduces the benefits of complementary medicine to the team, encourages self-care and promotes the holistic delivery of care to patients.
• Costs must be assessed and funding obtained prior to any meaningful complementary medicine service. Additional skills should be reflected in pay awards for nurses and equitable promotion opportunities maintained as for any other nursing skill and responsibility.

CONCLUSION

Cancer provokes anxiety. The subjective experience of the person experiencing cancer is not readily addressed by providers of health care, although cancer itself may be well treated. Nurses, especially cancer and palliative care nurses, have been at the forefront of attempts to soften the rigours of treatment, enhance the results of it and offer supportive therapies by providing complementary medicine. Costs in health care are being scrutinised and some local authorities recognise that a person who feels better will cost less than one who feels ill. Nurses provide an extremely cost-effective work force. Figures which establish cost-effectiveness of complementary therapy will promote their use. There are, however, many problems in attempting to use many of these interventions solely as techniques for symptom control. Instead there needs to be a focus on the wider social and therapeutic issues as well as the personal and professional ones which affect us as nurses.

The philosophies of complementary medicine, palliative care and holistic nursing share similar values and beliefs which make them natural team mates. Holistic nursing does not compromise any of the basic principles of complementary medicine. It cannot, however, be adopted without radical reassessment of usual practices. Such change occurs slowly and takes time to implement. The role of complementary medicine is being explored in efforts to provide an integrated public health service. Such a service must embrace the continuing biochemical, diagnostic and surgical advances with a wide range of therapeutic options from complementary medicine. Integration implies equal respect and partnership. Such attitudes will ensure that holistic principles are not subsumed by economic or political expediency and provide maximum benefit to patients. Health care professionals share the responsibility for ensuring that best practice is based on evidence that is qualitative and quantitative. The next two decades will see many changes in both the treatment of cancer and its delivery. I am hopeful that it will also provide a more powerful and nurturing service as well as a supportive environment for both patients and providers. Complementary medicine is a positive step forward, giving benefit to many, not least in the provision of comfort and hope.

REFERENCES

Arvigo R 1995 Satsun. Harper, San Francisco

Bannerman R H, Burton J, Ch'en W-C 1983 Traditional medicine and health care coverage. The World Health Organization, Geneva

British Medical Association 1993 Complementary medicine; new approaches to good practice. Oxford University Press, Oxford

Buckle J 1997 Clinical aromatherapy in nursing. Singular Publishing Group, San Diego

Buckman R, Sabbagh K 1994 Magic or medicine? an investigation into healing. Pan Books, London

Coward R 1989 The whole truth; the myth of alternative health. Faber & Faber, London

Davies B, Oberle K (1990) Dimensions of the supportive role of the nurse in palliative care. Oncology Nursing Forum 17:(1) 87–94

Eddy D 1994 In: Vincent C, Furnham A (eds) Complementary medicine: a research perspective. John Wiley, London

Estabrooks C 1989 Touch: a nursing strategy in the intensive care unit. Heart and Lung 18(4): 392–401

Estabrooks C, Morse J 1992 Toward a theory of touch: the touching process and acquiring a nursing style. Journal of Advanced Nursing 17: 448–456

Foundation for Integrated Medicine 1997 Integrated healthcare; a way forward for the next five years? FIM, London

Franchomme P 1980 Phytoguide; aromatherapy advanced therapy for infectious illness. International Phytomedical Foundation, France

Gamlin R D 1999 Sexuality: a challenge for nursing practice. Nursing Times 95(7): 48–51

Gerber R 1988 Vibrational medicine; new choices for healing ourselves. Bear & Co., New Mexico

Gillon R 1994 Medical ethics: four principles plus attention to scope. British Medical Journal 309: 184–188

Kienle G S, Kiene H 1998 The placebo effect: a scientific critique. Complementary Therapies in Medicine 6: 14–24

McCann K, McKenna H 1993 An examination of touch between nurses and elderly patients in a continuing care setting in Northern Ireland. Journal of Advanced Nursing 18: 838–846

McNamara P 1994 Massage for people with cancer. The Cancer Support Centre, Wandsworth

Macnish K 1998 An exploration of nursing touch: what is the role of touch for the palliative nurse specialist? Unpublished MSc thesis. The Institute of Cancer Research and Royal Marsden NHS Trust Library

Moore T 1992 Care of the soul; how to add depth and meaning to everyday life. Piatkus, London

Moyers B 1993 Healing and the mind. Harper Collins, London

NHS Confederation 1997 Complementary medicine in the NHS; managing the issues (research paper No 4). NHS Confederation, London

Payer L 1990 Medicine and culture: notions of sickness and health. Victor Gollancz, London

Pelletier K R 1977 Mind as healer, mind as slayer. Delta, New York

Pert C 1997 Molecules of emotion. Scribner, New York

Porter R 1997 The greatest benefit to mankind; a medical history of humanity from antiquity to the present. Harper Collins, London

Price S, Price L 1995 Aromatherapy for health care professionals. Churchill Livingstone, New York

Rankin-Box D 1997 Therapies in practice; survey assessing use of complementary therapies. Complementary Therapies in Nursing and Midwifery 3: 92–99

Select Committee on Medical Ethics 1994 Report on medical ethics 1994 (31/1/94). Government Select Committee, House of Commons, London

Talbot M 1991 The holographic universe. Harper Collins, New York

Tisserand R, Balacs T 1995 Essential oil safety: a guide for health care professionals. Churchill Livingstone, New York

Vithoulkas G 1980 The science of homeopathy. Grove Press, New York

Whitmont E C 1993 The alchemy of healing. North Atlantic Books, California

Wright S G 1995 Bringing the heart back into nursing. Complementary Therapies in Nursing and Midwifery 1(1): 15–20

Promoting hope through meaningful communication

8

Hope: an exploration of selected literature

Jacquelyn Chaplin
Rosemary McIntyre

INTRODUCTION

The study of hope could usefully be approached from a number of theoretical perspectives drawing on a rich literature from the knowledge base of psychology, theology, sociology or phenomenology. While acknowledging that unique and valuable insights could be gained by aligning this chapter with one of these specific fields of study, the authors have opted to adopt an eclectic stance. This broad-based approach should allow a range of theories to be accommodated in the discussion and will support an exploration of hope from a range of perspectives that includes both patients and relatives. The overriding priority will be to ensure relevance to palliative care practice.

The authors have a shared and enduring interest in the concept of hope in palliative care and the chapter reflects their combined backgrounds in cancer and palliative care research, education and practice. It should be noted that much of this chapter focuses on hope in adults with cancer, and does not directly explore hope in relation to other non-curative illnesses. This limitation is based upon the fact that much of the literature, and the authors' own research, involves patients and families experiencing a cancer illness. However readers are encouraged to reflect upon the relevance of the topics explored to individuals who are experiencing other non-curative progressive illnesses, such as motor neurone disease, auto- immune deficiency syndrome and chronic pulmonary disease.

McIntyre's doctoral action research study sought the views of nurses and relatives in the acute hospital setting to identify needs and concerns faced by the dying patient's family in the days leading up to the death and to explore difficulties experienced by nurses with this aspect of care. As part of this work, changes were implemented in the study wards, resulting in improved care and facilities for dying patients' families and in reduced distancing behaviour by nurses (McIntyre 1996, 1999).

Chaplin's background in cancer and palliative education and her masters' research work will also substantially inform the contents of this chapter. Chaplin's work used a case study approach and sought the perspectives of patients, relatives and nurses to explore the quality of care for patients undergoing surgery for lung cancer (Chaplin 1996).

Exemplars drawn from the authors' research findings are incorporated into Chapter 9 to illuminate particular experiences and issues and to give voice to those who receive palliative care. Steps have been taken to ensure the anonymity of the research participants.

In presenting this chapter the authors aim to present a literature-based analysis of hope which will allow readers to explore related concepts such as coping, denial and pretence. Chapter 8 will also provide readers with the foundation for subsequent analysis of the clinical relevance of this topic for palliative care. At various points in this chapter and in Chapter 9 the reader is encouraged to participate in activity arising from the literature, case studies and discussion of reflection on practice.

A REVIEW OF THE LITERATURE

Nurses often describe their feelings of helplessness when caring for an individual who appears to have given up hope, becomes increasingly withdrawn and who often quickly dies. Alternatively, nurses may have cared for patients who seem to be able to sustain hope despite circumstances which appear overwhelming.

Nowhere is this more apparent than in the field of palliative care where the strength of the human spirit is seriously challenged by the prospect of imminent death and yet, we often witness the personal growth of individuals who face this challenge. These reflections raise a number of questions. These include: What is hope? What relevance does the concept of hope have to palliative nursing care? How does hope relate to the individual's ability to cope with life-threatening illness? What can nurses do to foster hope in both patients and relatives within the context of palliative care?

HOPE DEFINED

Hope is a nebulous, elusive concept which has been variously defined in the psychological, sociological, theological and health care literature (Fromm 1968, Stotland 1969, Frankl 1984, Herth 1990). Hope has been described as being closely related to spiritual well-being in terms of providing a sense of meaning and purpose to life (Averill et al 1990). Hope has also been identified as an essential component of the unique human capacity to respond to adversity with the potential for personal growth and achievement (Carson et al 1988, Fehring et al 1997).

Hope and the dialectically opposed concept of hopelessness have also been explored in relation to the individual experience of suffering. An example of such work is research which focused on coping responses of concentration camp survivors in which survivors described hope as a kind of 'spiritual freedom' which gives life meaning and purpose (Frankl 1984). Alternatively, hopelessness, or the absence of hope, is associated with a loss of belief in the future and feelings of despair and powerlessness (Frankl 1984, Beck et al 1990). There is recognition that the dying experience can engender suffering and feelings of hopelessness in both the patient and family members (Longford 1990, Salt 1997). Indeed, there is evidence in the literature to suggest that the total absence of hope within an individual can produce a state of despair that can lead to inevitable death (Kubler-Ross 1969, Miller 1983, Hockley 1993).

A growing body of literature has examined the concept of hope in relation to people coping with illness and death (Herth 1990, Perakyla 1991, Stephenson 1991). The interest has now shifted from a focus on the role of hope in acute illnesses (O'Malley & Menke 1988, Cutcliffe 1996), to include hope in people affected by cancer (Herth 1989, 1991, Nowotny 1989, Hinds & Gattuso 1991, Post-White et al 1996) and in those experiencing non-curative illnesses (Herth 1990, Perakyla 1991, Flemming 1997).

While there is considerable debate regarding an accepted definition of hope, synthesis of the literature reveals that hope has a number of key characteristics. There is general acceptance that hope is multidimensional in character and dynamic in nature and that it provides an energising force which allows individuals to cope with their current life situation and also provides the opportunity for personal growth.

For the purposes of writing this chapter the authors have agreed to adopt the following definition as it represents a synthesis of the key attributes of the concept of hope that have emerged from the literature:

Hope is a dynamic inner power that enables transcendence of the present situation and fosters a positive new awareness of being.   (Herth 1993)

ATTRIBUTES OF HOPE

Farran et al (1995) offer an analysis of hope, where they describe hope as comprising four key attributes:

• *Hope as an experiential process* – the authors describe the experiential aspects of hope as ways of feeling that they refer to as the *pain* of hope.
• *Hope as a spiritual process* – this process is described as the *soul* of hope. In this context hope is influenced by a person's ways of thinking. The transcendental or spiritual process of hope is seen as being inseparable from faith in oneself and the future.
• *Hope as a rational process* – sometimes called the *mind* of hope. This describes the cognitive processes which enable alternative strategies to be identified for dealing with difficult situations within the context of the reality of that situation.
• *Hope as a relational process* – the final attribute, is inspired by love, evolves from relationships with others and is described by the authors as the *heart* of hope.

This description of the attributes of hope serves to demonstrate not only the complexity of this concept but also the complexity of human experience. The multidimensional nature of hope is further complicated by the fluid nature of hope and the way in which hope is influenced by the individual's life experiences.

A distinction has also been made between 'generalised unchallenged or fundamental hope' and 'challenged or particularised hope' (Dufault & Martocchio 1985, Scanlon 1989). Generalised or fundamental hope can be described as an enduring sense of 'positive inner strength' born out of previous personal, interpersonal and sociological experiences, where the use of successful strategies to cope with adversity sustains hope for the future. A generalised sense of hopefulness, therefore, provides the individual with a basis from which subsequent adversity may be faced and may help also provide a sense of purpose and meaning in life (Scanlon 1989).

On the other hand, challenged or particularised hope is a response to a particular perceived threat or adversity (Dufault & Martocchio 1985, Averill et al 1990). The notion of 'challenged hope' describes the common situation faced by people experiencing serious illness and those requiring palliative care. The physical, psychological, social and spiritual trauma experienced by people affected by advanced non-curative illness clearly can challenge an individual's capacity to maintain hope and may also profoundly influence the individual's search for meaning (O'Connor et al 1990, Ersek 1992). Challenged hope therefore is born out of both fundamental hope and the individual's response to adversity. It is dynamic in nature and is clearly related to the individual's capacity to cope. This relationship will be explored further in a later section.

The changing nature of any illness means that maintaining hope in the individual is a process requiring ongoing adaptation and flexibility (Cutcliffe 1995). Perakyla (1991) confirmed the fluctuating levels of hope reported by patients in a leukaemia ward where initially hope was focused on cure and survival. The fluctuating and dynamic nature of hope within the context of palliative care has also been widely reported (Hockley 1993, Flemming 1997, Brant 1998). A feature of this dynamic process is the repeated fluctuation that can occur between hope and hopelessness (Beck et al 1990, Farran & Popovich 1990). Herth (1993) offers a powerful image of hope when she describes hope in terms of a 'continually unfolding and changing in response to life's situations'. An important point to remember for those caring for individuals requiring palliative care is that hope can be influenced not only by the individual himself but also by other people (Carson et al 1988, Hinds 1988).

It is important that hope is differentiated from the related but different concepts of wishing and optimism. Wishing and optimism are more inflexible and focused in character than hope. Accordingly, they may actually limit how effectively an individual copes with a situation (Peterson & Bossio 1991). However, the role of wishing and optimism in supporting an individual to a more hopeful stance is still unclear. It has been suggested that the wishing is more superstitious than hope, and as such is often unrealistic (Peterson & Bossio 1991, Farran et al 1995).

FACTORS INFLUENCING HOPE

A range of factors influence hope in a person facing non-curative illness. These can be sociological, psychological, physical or spiritual in nature. It has already been stated that foundational or generalised hope is partly derived from developmental processes and is born out of the love of others with whom we have close or important relationships (Erikson 1982). Consequently, variations in generalised hope may be socially derived and may influence how an individual copes with dying. In addition, different care settings and social contexts may influence the sustenance of hope within the dying person and the family (Herth 1993, Nekolaichuk & Bruera 1998). Further research in this area is required.

Furthermore, the effect that positive relationships with others can have on levels of hope has been reported by a number of authors (Scanlon 1989, Herth 1990, Hockley 1993, Post-White et al 1996). In particular, Scanlon graphically describes the interactional nature of hope by describing hope as a 'contagious reality' (Scanlon 1989). The interactional quality of hope is explored in more detail in the next chapter as the nurse–patient relationship, patient–relative relationship and nurse–relative relationship are all fundamental to fostering hope within the context of palliative care.

Physical factors have also been found to influence hope. In a small-scale qualitative study Flemming (1997) explored the meaning of hope for patients in a palliative care unit. Flemming found that patients placed importance on maintaining their physical condition and they identified clear links between physical comfort and the sustenance of hope. Moreover, the physical, emotional and psychological disengagement which often precedes death may also have an impact upon the hope of the family, causing them to dismantle any residual hope of recovery and accept the reality of the impending death (Scanlon 1989). A number of authors have highlighted the relationship between hope and coping (Scanlon 1989, McIntyre 1996, Fehring et al 1997, Chapman & Pepler 1998). Before going on to explore the relationship between hope and coping first consider what relevance the above literature has for your own area of practice.

Reflection point

- Think of a patient for whom you have provided palliative care.
- Consider whether and how hope altered for that individual and the family during the course of the illness.
- What factors influenced your patient's levels of hopefulness?
- What factors influenced the relatives' level of hopefulness?

HOPE AND COPING

The literature, so far described, confirms that hope is a multifaceted concept with theoretical roots grounded in a range of knowledge bases and related disciplines. When considering hope's main dimensions, striking parallels emerge between stress and coping theory and the hope literature. This is particularly apparent when exploring the experiences of people affected by incurable illness.

Within this context the intricate relationship between stress and hope is clear. This relationship is of an inverse nature, in that severe unremitting stress, such as that encountered in terminal illness, severely taxes the capacity for hope for those involved (McIntyre 1996). Moreover, evidence from the literature that identifies factors found to influence and support coping during a fatal illness closely mirrors the factors cited in the hope literature as having 'hope facilitating' qualities (Herth 1993, McIntyre 1996).

To illustrate the congruence of the theoretical perspectives of the hope and coping literature, a brief overview will be offered of stress and coping theory. In examining this related body of literature it is intended that the links to hope will become apparent. In Chapter 9 a more detailed exploration of specific links between hope and denial is offered when addressing issues affecting relatives of dying patients.

Coping styles and strategies

Coping represents a complex ongoing struggle involving a whole constellation of processes aimed at countering the stress. The main aims of coping are to take steps to (a) manage the stressful situation (problem-focused coping) and (b) to regulate feelings of distress which arise from such situations (emotion-focused coping) (Lazarus & Folkman 1984).

Problem-focused coping

Problem-focused coping usually involves positive action and is only possible in situations where there is potential to eliminate, modify or control the source of the stress (Lazarus & Folkman 1984). The coping response which is generated will be based on the individual's subjective appraisal of the threat they believe they are facing and the potential that they

judge that this has for amelioration. When problem-solving efforts are deemed pointless, then emotion-focused approaches might offer the only appropriate coping response (Wrubel et al 1981).

Emotion-focused coping

Emotion-focused coping aims to alter perceptions of a situation in order to reduce the degree of threat it presents and to regulate the distressing emotions it generates. Clarke calls this 'indirect' or 'palliative' coping (Clarke 1984), while more than 20 years ago Lazarus used the term 'cognitive coping' (Lazarus 1976). Cognitive coping encompasses a range of psychological defence mechanisms, which include denial and avoidance. Such mechanisms can operate in a protective fashion to allow the individual to control the emotional impact of stressful situations.

Research confirms that problem-focused and emotion-focused coping responses tend to be used synchronously by most people in managing stress (Pearlin & Schooler 1978, Folkman 1984).

Influences on coping

Within every stressful encounter, dynamic and reciprocal factors operate and the coping efforts that result tend to occur within this transactional context. Factors that influence coping arise from a range of sources originating within (a) the situation, (b) the environment and (c) the person. Each will briefly be considered and links to hope will be suggested.

Factors within the situation

In the situation of impending loss, feelings of helplessness and loss of control may render the individual vulnerable to stress and breakdown (Wrubel et al 1981). Situations which are unremitting in character can severely tax coping resources, leading to exhaustion and hopelessness. Protracted illness is precisely this sort of situation which, because of its unrelenting nature, challenges the capacity for hope. Finally, situations which are ambiguous and unpredictable, as can be experienced in advanced illness, are generally perceived as being highly challenging (Benner & Wrubel 1989).

Factors within the environment

The literature confirms that, where events might be experienced by patients and relatives as alien and unpredictable, stress can be generated by a perceived lack of information (Steptoe & Sutcliffe 1991). The situation is not, however, entirely clear. While there is substantial evidence to indicate that for most people information provides a sense of personal efficacy and control, for others it might threaten cognitive coping mechanisms such as denial (Steptoe & Sutcliffe 1991). As individuals will, to some extent, exercise choice in the extent to which they seek, use or reject information as a coping resource, the provision of information should not preclude the use of denial and other avoidance strategies (Janis 1983, Fallowfield 1993). Hospice care, while different from the acute setting, may also be stressful for some individuals. In this situation, stress may arise from preconceptions of the role of hospices in health care and the association such institutions have with death and suffering.

Supportive social relationships including family, friends and co-workers also influence profoundly coping effectiveness (Nugent 1988, McIntyre 1996). This has important implications for supporting coping during terminal illness. As close family members normally represent the patient's primary source of support, by ensuring that relatives are made welcome and comfortable in the ward, nurses may contribute to facilitating comfort and hope in the dying patient (McIntyre 1996).

Factors within the person

The literature offers convincing evidence that many, though not all, people exposed to severe sustained stress, such as that experienced by relatives during an incurable illness in a loved one, exhibit physical and psychiatric ill health (Nixon 1993, Larsson et al 1994, McGhee 1994).

To explore the complex range of factors which help people cope with potentially devastating circumstances, Antonovsky (1987) reported on studies of stress in survivors of the holocaust. He noted that some people, despite having been subjected to significant stress, appeared to suffer no lasting physical or psychological damage. This led him to question 'whence the strength?' and drove him to explore the phenomenon of 'salutogenesis'.

Salutogenesis refers to the apparent resistance which some individuals exhibit to developing stress-induced pathology. Salutogenesis can be contrasted with 'pathogenesis', where physiological and/or psychological harm results from stress (Strumpfer 1990). Antonovsky suggests those people who had 'survived' stress apparently unscathed had been able to call on a whole range of resources, including physiological, economic, cognitive, emotional, interpersonal and cultural resources to support them and to protect them against the effects of stress. These were described as 'general resistance resources' which, when combined with a successful coping history, appeared to provide a personal 'sense of coherence' (Antonovsky 1987).

'Sense of coherence' is associated with a personality orientation that views one's environment as predictable and controllable and believes that coping resources are available to meet demands. People with a strong sense of coherence tend to view demands as positive challenges and are by disposition 'fundamentally hopeful'. Parallels between Antonovsky's concept of sense of coherence and high fundamental levels of hopefulness are striking. Post-White et al (1996), researching the meaning of hope in adult cancer patients, found a clear relationship between sense of coherence and hope.

It has also been suggested that an individual's sense of coherence, and capacity for hope, can be strengthened by an approach to care that is supportive, reduces uncertainty and enhances the personal feelings of control (Herth 1990, 1993, McIntyre 1996).

Kobasa (1979) also studied the impact of stress on health. Like Antonovsky, he found that while some people exhibited symptoms of ill health when exposed to stress others stayed well (Kobasa 1979). Kobasa attributed this apparent resilience to a quality described as 'personality hardiness'. Characteristics of personality hardiness include a clear sense of self; an understanding of one's personal values, goals and capabilities; a good degree of social involvement; and an internal locus of control. It is suggested that people with 'hardy personalities' tend to view change as a normal part of life which offers opportunities for personal growth (Leefarr & Cutler 1994).

People with an internal locus of control view themselves as active agents who are self-directing and able to exercise some control over events that affect them. Conversely, those with an external locus of control believe events to be outwith their control and see their fate as being largely determined by external forces (Rotter 1966). Perception of self as a helpless victim in the face of uncontrollable events diminishes the individual's sense of hope and purpose in living (Post-White et al 1996).

Notions of personal control and mastery are central to Antonovsky's 'sense of coherence', Kobasa's 'personality hardiness' and Rotter's 'locus of control'. Control and mastery appear to exert a positive influence on coping outcomes and, in salutogenic terms, result in reduced psychological or physical ill health arising from stressful encounters (Antonovsky 1987).

The relevance of these concepts to palliative care practice is worthy of sensitive debate. Palliative care nurses might usefully ponder on observations that patients who seem best able to cope with the difficulties they confront are often also those who display a fundamental capacity for hopefulness and who seem to approach their own dying showing evidence of personal growth. Nurses must be very careful not to make value judgements about the responses of others who are facing the profound and ultimate challenge of impending death.

Terminal illness generates considerable distress and vulnerability in the patient and family. By offering information and supportive physical and emotional care it should be possible to enhance their sense of control and mastery and to decrease feelings of powerlessness, alienation and hopelessness (Steptoe & Sutcliffe 1991). Facilitating hope should then be a realistic goal.

MEASURING HOPE

The literature reviewed above demonstrates the relationship of hope to coping and the relevance of hope and coping theory to palliative nursing. Increasingly, nurse researchers have been examining the relationship of hope to health and illness. In an attempt to understand the meaning of hope in malignant disease, hope and adolescents with cancer (Hinds 1988) and hope and adults with cancer has been explored (Ersek 1992, Raleigh 1992, El-Gamel 1993, Post-White et al 1996, Ballard et al 1997).

Different perspectives on hope have also been examined. These include hope in palliative and terminal care patients (Herth 1993, Flemming 1997); hope from the perspective of the family (Herth 1993, Chapman & Pepler 1998); and hope from the perspective of the nurses caring for patients with cancer and other terminal illnesses (Cutcliffe 1995, Koopmeiners et al 1997, Benzein & Saveman 1998).

While some research has been focused on understanding the concept of hope, other studies have attempted to measure hope. As a result of this work a number of tools have been developed to help with the measurement of hope in different populations.

As will be seen from Table 8.1, a considerable range of tools have now been developed to measure hope. However, issues arising from their potential use in measuring hope in those receiving palliative nursing care require to be carefully evaluated and debated.

The contribution of hope measurement tools to the practice of palliative care can be questioned on a number of counts. Many of the tools are time and energy demanding to complete, some having up to 60 self-report items in a questionnaire format. The physical demands that this can place on already stressed patients, even when given assistance to complete them, means

Table 8.1 Measurement of hope

Hope measurement tool	Population studied	Approach	Dimensions
Gottschalk Hope Scale (Gottschalk 1974)	Healthy adults and psychologically impaired adults and adolescents	Interview content analysis	Multidimensional: focuses on feelings of hope for present and future
The Hope Scale (Erickson et al 1975)	Psychiatric patients	30-item goal oriented statements	Unidimensional: probability of goal attainment
The Hope Index Scale (Obayuwana et al 1982)	Psychiatric patients	60-item dichotomous Yes/No questionnaire	Multidimensional: ego strength, religion, perceived human/family support, education and economic assets
Miller Hope Scale (Miller & Powers 1988)	Healthy adults	40-item 5-point Likert scale	Multidimensional: *including*: affiliation, sense of possible, achieving goals, meaning in life, optimum mental and physical ability
Stoner Hope Scale (Stoner 1988)	Adult cancer patients	20-item questionnaire	Unidimensional: assesses importance of and probability of goal attainment
Herth Hope Scale (Herth 1989)	Healthy elderly adults and adult cancer patients	30-item 4-point Likert scale	Multidimensional: cognitive, affective and affiliative
Hope Index (Staats 1989)	Elderly healthy adults	16-item questionnaires	Unidimensional: assesses 16-goal statements related to self and external factors
Nowotny Hope Scale (Nowotny 1989)	Healthy adults and adults with cancer	29-item 4-point Likert scale focusing on a stressful event	Multidimensional: confidence in outcome, relates to others, future is possible, spiritual beliefs, involvement and inner readiness
Hopefulness Scale for Adolescents (Hinds & Gattuso 1991)	Healthy adolescents, adolescents with mental disturbances, adolescents with cancer	24-item visual analogue scale	Unidimensional: degree of positive future orientation
Snyder Hope Scale (Snyder et al 1991)	Healthy adults (children's version Kid Hope Scale)	8-item 4-point Likert scale	Unidimensional: cognitive appraisal of ability to achieve goals
Herth Hope Index (Herth 1992)	Acutely ill, clinically ill, terminally ill adults	Adaptation of HHS for clinical use 12-item 4-point Likert scale	Multidimensional: spiritual, rational, relational

that many are unsuitable for palliative care patients or may be suitable only at an earlier point in the dying process. An exception is the 12-item Herth Hope Index specifically developed for use in the palliative care clinical setting and with terminally ill patients (Herth 1992). The Herth Hope Index has been used extensively in the United States (Farran et al 1995).

However, there is little evidence of its use in the United Kingdom in palliative care, although it has been found to be practical and clinically relevant when used with oncology patients (El-Gamel 1993).

Furthermore, it is not clear when and where such tools should be used. Little is known about how levels of hope fluctuate during the course of the terminal illness. Consequently, the usefulness of using a particular tool to measure hope at one point in time remains unclear. Nor is it known whether a tool tested in one care setting may be appropriate in others, e.g. acute hospital, community or hospice setting.

Another crucial factor is that the multidimensional nature of hope, and the differing theoretical frameworks upon which the tools are based, need to be understood when evaluating the usefulness of a hope measurement tool for a particular client group (Klyma & Vehvilainen-Julkunen 1997).

This raises the question: Is it possible that palliative care nurses might run the risk of losing the holistic approach by attempting to obtain hard empirical data to measure hope, some of which lacks clinical utility? This closely reflects the debate surrounding quality of life measurement tools as applied within palliative care where it is suggested that a more patient-centred individualistic approach is required. To support palliative care nursing practice, more clinically relevant hope measurement tools need to be developed and tested by research.

CONCLUSION

The literature reviewed in this section has revealed hope in some of its complexity and has confirmed that it presents a challenge to nurses. This is especially so for nurses who provide palliative care. There is evidence that hope is multidimensional in nature, fluctuating in character and is closely related to coping. Many factors influence hope, especially human relationships. The literature confirms that while a number of attempts have been made to research hope in palliative care, little is still known about how the focus of hope changes during the course of the terminal illness for both the patient and the relatives. If nurses accept that hope is an essential component of human existence then as carers of people near the end of their existence, understanding of the concept of hope is fundamental to holistic palliative care. Chapter 9 explores the concept of hope in relation to palliative care in more detail. Before reading the next chapter the reader may find it useful to consider the relevance of the issues arising from the literature to his/her own area of practice.

REFERENCES

Antonovsky A 1987 Unravelling the mystery of health; how people manage stress and stay well. Jossey-Bass, San Francisco

Averill J R, Catlin G, Chon K K 1990 Rules of hope. Springer-Verlag, New York

Ballard A, Green T, McCarr A, Logsdon M 1997 A comparison of the level of hope in patients with newly diagnosed and recurrent cancer. Oncology Nursing Forum 24(5): 899–904

Beck A, Brown G, Berchick R J, Stewart B L, Steer R A 1990 Relationships between hopelessness and ultimate suicide. American Journal of Psychiatry 147(2): 190–195

Benner P E, Wrubel J 1989 The primacy of caring: stress and coping in health and illness. Addison-Wesley Publishing Company, California

Benzein E, Saveman B 1998 Nurses' perception of hope in patients with cancer: a palliative care perspective. Cancer Nursing 21(1): 10–16

Brant J M 1998 The art of palliative care: living with hope, dying with dignity. Oncology Nursing Forum 25(6): 995–1004

Carson V, Soeken K L, Grimm R M 1988 Hope and its relationship to spiritual well-being. Journal of Psychology and Theology 16: 159–167

Chaplin J 1996 An exploration of the quality of care received by individuals having lung cancer surgery: perceptions of patients, relatives and nurses. Dissertation, University of Glasgow

Chapman K J, Pepler C 1998 Coping, hope and anticipatory grief in family members in palliative home care. Cancer Nursing 21(4): 226–234

Clarke M 1984 Stress and coping: constructs for nursing. Journal of Advanced Nursing 9: 3–13

Cutcliffe J R 1995 How do nurses inspire and instil hope in terminally ill HIV patients? Journal of Advanced Nursing 22: 888–895

Cutcliffe J 1996 Critically ill patients' perspectives of hope. British Journal of Nursing 5(11): 674, 687–690

Dufault K, Martocchio B 1985 Hope: its spheres and dimensions. Nursing Clinics of North America 20(2): 379–391

El-Gamel V A 1993 The usefulness of hope for a nursing assessment on the oncology unit. Journal of Cancer Care 2: 22–30

Erickson E, Post R, Paige A 1975 Hope as a psychiatric variable. Journal of Clinical Psychology 31: 324–330

Erikson E H 1982 The life cycle completed: a review. Norton, New York

Ersek M 1992 The process of maintaining hope in adults undergoing bone marrow transplantation. Oncology Nursing Forum 19(6): 883–889

Fallowfield L 1993 Evaluation of counselling in the National Health Service. Journal of the Royal Society of Medicine 86(7): 429–430

Farran C J, Popovitch J 1990 Hope: a relevant concept for geriatric psychiatry. Archives in Psychiatric Nursing 4: 127–130

Farran C J, Herth K, Popovitch J M 1995 Hope and hopelessness: critical clinical constructs. Sage Publications, Thousand Oaks

Fehring R J, Miller J F, Shaw C 1997 Spiritual well-being, religiosity, hope, depression, and other mood states in elderly people coping with cancer. Oncology Nursing Forum 24(4): 663–671

Flemming K 1997 The meaning of hope to palliative care cancer patients. International Journal of Palliative Nursing 3(1): 14–18

Folkman S 1984 Personal control and stress and coping processes: a theoretical analysis. Journal of Personality and Social Psychology 46(4): 839–852

Frankl V E 1984 Man's search for meaning. Washington Square, New York

Fromm E 1968 The revolution of hope. Harper & Row, New York

Gottschalk 1 1974 A hope scale applicable to verbal samples. Archives of General Psychiatry 30: 779–785

Herth K A 1989 The relationship between level of hope and level of coping response and other variables in patients with cancer. Oncology Nursing Forum 16(1): 67–72

Herth K A 1990 Fostering hope in terminally ill people. Journal of Advanced Nursing 15: 1250–1259

Herth K 1991 Development and refinement of an instrument to measure hope. Scholarly Inquiry for Nursing Practice 5(1): 39–51

Herth K A 1992 An abbreviated instrument to measure hope: development and psychometric evaluation. Journal of Advanced Nursing 17: 1251–1259

Herth K A 1993 Hope in the family caregiver of terminally ill people. Journal of Advanced Nursing 18: 538–548

Hinds P 1988 Adolescent hopefulness in illness and health. Advances in Nursing Science 10: 79–88

Hinds P, Gattuso J 1991 Measuring hopefulness in adolescents. Journal of Paediatric Oncology 8(2): 92–94

Hockley J 1993 The concept of hope and the will to live. Palliative Medicine 7: 181–186

Janis I L 1983 Stress inoculation in health care; theory and research. In: Meichelbaum D J (ed.) Stress reduction and reduction. Plenum Press, New York

Klyma J, Vehvilainen-Julkunen K 1997 Hope in nursing research: a meta-analysis of the ontological and epistemological foundations of research on hope. Journal of Advanced Nursing 25: 364–371

Kobasa S 1979 Stressful life events; personality and health; an inquiry into hardiness. In: Strumpfer D J W (1990) Salutogenesis: a new paradigm: South African Journal of Psychology 24(4): 265–276

Koopmeiners L, Post-White J, Gutknecht S et al 1997 How healthcare professionals contribute to hope in patients with cancer. Oncology Nursing Forum 24(9): 1507–1513

Kubler-Ross E 1969 On death and dying. Macmillan, New York

Larsson G, Kallenberg K, Setterlind S, Starrin B 1994 Health and loss of a family member; impact on sense of coherence. International Journal of Health Sciences 5(1): 5–11

Lazarus R, Folkman S 1984 Stress, appraisal and coping. Springer Verlag, New York

Lazarus R S 1976 Patterns of adjustment. McGraw-Hill, New York

Leefarr V, Cutler M 1994 Stress. In: Alexander M, Fawcet J, Runciman P (eds) Nursing practice hospital and home. The adult. Churchill Livingstone, Edinburgh, pp. 575–596

Longford B 1990 Suffering and hope. Collins, London

McGhee M 1994 The impact of grief. Update June: 9089–9110

McIntyre R 1996 Nursing support for relatives of dying cancer patients in hospital: Improving standards by research. Doctoral Thesis, Glasgow Caledonian University

McIntyre R 1999 The family in focus. In: Lugton J, Kindlen M (eds) Palliative care: the nursing role. Harcourt Brace, Edinburgh

Miller J F 1983 Coping with chronic illness: overcoming powerlessness. F A Davis, Philadelphia

Miller J F, Powers M 1988 Development of an instrument to measure hope. Nursing Research 37(1): 6–10

Nekolaichuk C L, Bruera E 1998 On the nature of hope in palliative care. Journal of Palliative Care 14(1): 36–42

Nixon P 1993 The broken heart – counteraction by SABRES. Journal of the Royal Society of Medicine 86(8): 468–471

Nowotny M 1989 Assessment of hope in patients with cancer: development of an instrument. Oncology Nursing Forum 16(1): 75–79

Nugent L S 1998 The social support requirements of family caregivers of terminal cancer patients. Canadian Journal of Nursing Research 20(3): 45–58

O'Connor A P, Wicker C A, Germino B B 1990 Understanding the cancer patient's search for meaning. Cancer Nursing 13: 167–175

O'Malley P, Menke E 1988 Relationship of hope and stress after M.I. Heart and Lung 17(2): 184–190

Obayuwana A, Collins J, Carter A, Rao M, Mathura C, Wilson S 1982 Hope Index Scale: an instrument for objective assessment of hope. Journal of the National Medical Association 74(8): 761–765

Pearlin L, Schooler C 1978 The structure of coping. Journal of Health and Social Behaviour 19(March): 2–21

Perakyla A 1991 Hope work in the care of seriously ill patients. Qualitative Health Research 1(4): 407–433

Peterson C, Bossio I M 1991 Health and optimism. Free Press, New York

Post-White J, Ceronsky C, Kreitzer M J et al 1996 Hope, spirituality, sense of coherence, and quality of life in patients with cancer. Oncology Nursing Forum 23(10): 1571–1578

Raleigh E 1992 Sources of hope in chronic illness. Oncology Nursing Forum 19(3): 443–448

Rotter J B 1966 Generalised expectancies for internal versus external locus of control. In: Strumpfer D J W 1990 Salutogenesis: a new paradigm. South African Journal of Psychology 20(4): 265–276

Salt S 1997 Towards a definition of suffering. European Journal of Palliative Care 4(2): 58–60

Scanlon C 1989 Creating a vision of hope: the challenge of palliative care. Oncology Nursing Forum 16(4): 491–496

Snyder C, Harris C, Anderson J et al 1991 The will and the ways: development and validation of an individual-differences measure of hope. Journal of Personality and Social Psychology 60(4): 570–585

Staats S 1989 A comparison of two self-report measures for adults. Journal of Personality Assessment 53(2): 366–375

Stephenson C 1991 The concept of hope revisited for nursing. Journal of Advanced Nursing 16: 1456–1461

Steptoe A, Sutcliffe I 1991 Satisfaction with communication, medical knowledge, and coping style in patients with metastatic cancer. Social Science & Medicine 32(6): 627–632

Stoner M 1988 Measuring hope. In: Stromborg M (ed.) Instruments for clinical nursing practice. Appleton & Lange, Norwalk, CT, pp. 133–140

Stotland E 1969 The psychology of hope. Jossey-Bass, San Francisco

Strumpfer D 1990 Salutogenesis: a new paradigm. South African Journal of Psychology 20(4): 265–276

Wrubel J, Benner P, Lazarus R S 1981 Social competence from the perspective of stress and coping. In: Wine J, Smye M (eds) Social competence. The Guilford Press, New York, pp. 61–99

9

Hope: the heart of palliative care

Rosemary McIntyre
Jacquelyn Chaplin

INTRODUCTION

Having provided a literature-based analysis of hope in Chapter 8 the authors will now focus on ways in which hope is experienced within the context of palliative care practice. In presenting this chapter the authors aim to utilise insights gained from literature, research and practice to inform an analysis of hope as it relates to palliative care. Key and interrelated themes will also be described and used as a framework to analyse the experience of hope within incurable advanced illness. Insights gained will be used to explore the experience of hope within advanced illness and propose interventions aimed at promoting and supporting hope in both patients and relatives.

The authors would like to tentatively offer a conceptual model of hope as a vehicle for exploring the hope-related experiences of patients and relatives and as a framework for proposing hope-sustaining interventions.

Based on the key themes 'comfort', 'attachment' and 'worth', the model is designed to be simple, practical, but inclusive enough to offer readers a framework for reflecting on issues arising from the literature and from their practices. The origins of this simple model lie in the literature and in the research work of both authors (Chaplin 1996, McIntyre 1996). In particular, the themes offer a distillation of the factors found by McIntyre to relieve distress in relatives and factors found by Herth to foster hope in dying patients and in their relatives (Herth 1990, 1993).

A CONCEPTUAL MODEL OF HOPE

In this chapter the authors will utilise their conceptual model to explore the concept of hope as experienced by patients and relatives within the context of palliative care. This model incorporates three key themes: comfort, worth and attachment.

The three key themes of hope are comfort, attachment and worth. Figure 9.1 demonstrates the interrelationship of the key themes. The themes are not only interrelated but are also dynamic, complex and potentially synergistic in nature. In turn, each theme is affected by a range of factors which will affect the experience.

Figure 9.1 identifies the three key themes and illustrates the negative and positive parameters of each theme. More difficult to represent in this format is the interconnectedness of the themes and the transactional relationship that operates between the themes – in that factors found to impact on one theme will have a reciprocal effect on the other themes.

It is intended that the model will allow opposite, yet related, constructs related to each of the key themes, to be located on a continuum in terms of their 'hope-sustaining' or 'hope-diminishing' potential.

In the section which follows each theme will be explored in relation to the patient's experience of palliative care. Implications for practice and the potential for sustaining or diminishing hope in patients facing incurable illness will be considered. A similar thematic exploration of the experience of close relatives of dying patients will

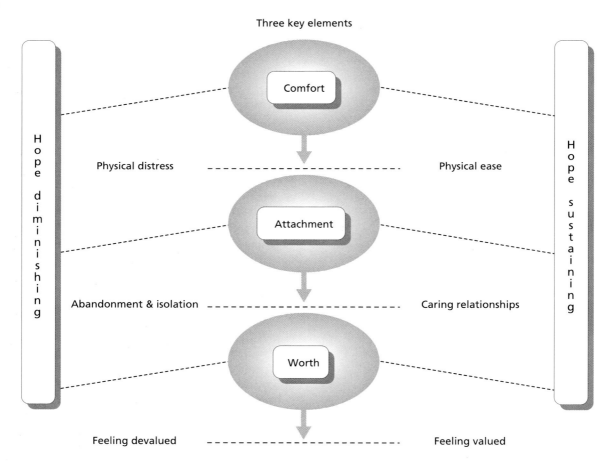

Figure 9.1 Interrelationships of the three key themes.

follow. The particular focus is on identifying hope-sustaining interventions.

The same approach will be applied to an analysis of research-based examplars and case studies. The reader will be encouraged to utilise the framework to reflect on, and evaluate, their own practice in terms of its capacity to nurture and support hope in patients and relatives experiencing palliative care.

THE PATIENT'S EXPERIENCE OF HOPE

A person who is required to confront the reality of his own dying will experience many challenges to his capacity to sustain hope (Flemming 1997). Advancing disease, diminished physical functioning and the social and emotional impact of terminal illness can all contribute to an experience in which hope may appear to be lost or given up (Hockley 1993).

It is intended that the conceptual framework used in this chapter will facilitate an inclusive and holistic approach to support an exploration of the complex issues surrounding hope in palliative care, and will also assist in identifying and avoiding hope-diminishing situations, and in providing hope-sustaining interventions.

THEME 1: COMFORT

Physical distress . . . . Physical ease

Pain and other symptoms are commonly experienced in the last years and months of life in advanced malignancy. Pain has long been recognised as having psychological, spiritual and social as well as physical dimensions (Saunders 1984). As such, pain and other symptoms have a multidimensional impact on the individual who experiences them (Post-White et al 1996, Flemming 1997).

Case study 9.1 illustrates the complexities of providing high-quality palliative care that is truly holistic in approach and that recognises and addresses the challenges to hope which such situations present.

Comment on Case study 9.1

Sadie's symptoms threaten her capacity for hope in a number of ways. Pain, and suffering due to

---

CASE STUDY 9.1

SADIE'S STORY

Sadie is a 43-year-old married mother of two with advanced apical lung cancer. She experienced severe pain which was poorly controlled initially while she was nursed at home. This was a very difficult time for Sadie, who became very withdrawn yet at the same time acutely anxious. Eventually the pain was identified as being neuropathic in nature and was eventually controlled by amitriptyline. Later in her illness Sadie experienced a spinal cord compression due to spinal metastases which responded partially to steroids and radiotherapy. Sadie's backache resolved, but she continued to experience urinary and faecal incontinence. In the last few weeks of her life she was cared for at home by her family with support from the primary health care team.

---

other symptoms, challenge her ability to cope with her illness experience. Sadie's experience, which is multidimensional in its nature, generated fears and concerns for the future. These fears included uncertainties regarding the future severity of the pain and other symptoms, and concerns about her capacity to cope in the future.

Difficulties in controlling Sadie's neuropathic pain because of the pain's resistance to opioids made Sadie fearful for the future and thus diminished her levels of hope. Sadie had coped with this by focusing on her children's needs until the pain became so severe that this was no longer effective. This was manifested by her withdrawal and introspection. Sadie's primary desire was to stay at home with her children for as long as possible – yet the uncontrolled pain threatened this.

Another key factor was Sadie's confidence in the health care professionals' abilities to control her symptoms. Sadie was fearful, born out of her experiences, that greater pain was ahead and she was concerned that it would not be effectively managed by her GP in whom she had lost trust.

The final stages of progressive non-curative illnesses often include diminishing control over body functions. Increased fatigue and muscle weakness associated with many illnesses – cancer, motor neurone disease, end-stage cardiac failure, etc. – result in individuals affected by these illnesses having to come to terms with the

Another aspect of this theme of worth is the need for individuals to feel autonomous as people and to have a sense of meaning and purpose in life. One of the dilemmas for nurses is that sometimes, in the provision of caring for the dying, nurses run the risk of taking over and organising people's lives in the name of caring. Many decisions are made by professionals and family members caring for the person who is dying, e.g. who should visit, medication, when to get out of bed, where to die. However, this lack of autonomous decision making can have a profound devaluing effect on the person with advanced disease whose sense of personal control may already be threatened by the disease process itself.

In addition, it has been recognised that hope is enhanced if the individual feels able to die at peace with their inner self. Many elderly people die at peace because they feel they have lived their life fully, have put their affairs in order and are ready to say goodbye. This acceptance of death is a positive action which surprisingly sustains hope, whereas having 'unfinished business' may detract from the individual's ability to move on. Kubler-Ross (1969) described the acceptance of death in an attempt to understand the psychological stages involved in the process of dying. The concept of this adaptive process being in stages is often criticised. Therefore, the professional's acceptance of the individuality of the person's response to the loss of self which they are experiencing as part of the dying process is crucial in fostering self-worth. Recognition by health care professionals that the aspects of loss in terminal illness – denial, anger, bargaining, depression and acceptance – can be experienced in a truly individualistic way rather than in sequential stages is important to support the person's feelings of personal worth.

Another factor influencing hope is the individual's sense of a personal future. In haematology/oncology patients the sense of a personal future which is a factor in the sustenance of hope is firmly linked to hope for survival (Perakyla 1991, Post-White et al 1996). In a palliative care context the sense of a personal future is not necessarily focused on a physical future. It is related to three aspects: the affirmation of what one has been; that the knowledge that opportunities still exist to live life meaningfully; and a belief that one will 'live on' after physical death.

Confirmation of self-worth can often be achieved by review of what has been (Lair 1996). Nurses who care for people who are dying will recognise that, commonly, patients feel the need to talk about their life. This life review can be very beneficial to the patient, reaffirming their self-value and allowing them the opportunity to put death into the perspective of living.

The concept of providing support to ensure the opportunity to live life fully until death occurs is fundamental to palliative care (de Raeve 1996). The belief that good days, happy times or meaningful moments can be enjoyed can only be supported through the provision of holistic palliative care, symptom management, emotional support, financial and physical care, and family care.

Furthermore, the belief that as an individual one is able to 'live on' in the memories of others or that a bit of 'self' lives on in children and grandchildren can be a positive supporter of hope. Family members can be encouraged to contribute positively to the patient's hope by reminiscing and remembering family memories. Individuals may also find support for hope in religious beliefs which may encompass faith in spiritual life after death. Again, the nurse can play a key role in supporting the individual religious beliefs of both the patients and family.

NURTURING HOPE

A range of interventions have been identified which nurture hope in patients receiving palliative care (Table 9.1). These interventions are intended as a guide and are not considered to be all inclusive. A key aspect of nurturing hope is that interventions are potentially synergistic in nature and, while discussed individually, the holistic nature of palliative care requires that an integrated approach be adopted.

The interrelatedness of all these themes cannot be overstressed. The following interventions are offered as ways in which palliative care nurses can nurture hope in their patients.

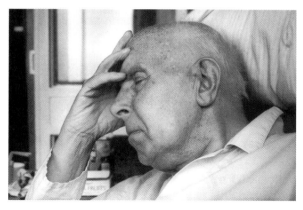

Figure 9.2   Duncan: photograph by Colin Dickson from the exhibition 'Remaining Human: Photographs of People with Cancer', reproduced with kind permission of the photographer and the patient/family.

HOPE IN RELATIVES

Review of key themes

The key themes in the model of hope offered in this chapter will now be related to relatives who are facing the death of a close family member. It should be noted that the term 'relative' or 'family' will refer to the person or persons who have an enduring emotional attachment to the patient, and who share the patient's experience of palliative care. This definition will apply whether kinship links exist or not.

Review of the themes comfort, attachment and worth will be approached in a number of ways.

Reflection point 9A

Consider a patient you have cared for recently who has advanced cancer:

- Which of the interventions in Table 9.1 were employed to nurture that person's sense of hope?
- Were any of these interventions not utilised?
- If so, how could they be implemented in the future?

  Now consider a patient with advanced non-malignant disease.

- Are the interventions in Table 9.1 relevant?

What, if any, difficulties arise in the implementation of these interventions for either patients with advanced malignant disease or patients with non-malignant disease?

Table 9.1   Hope-nurturing interventions in palliative care

Theme	Interventions	Rationale
Comfort Aim: to promote physical ease	• Comprehensively assess/regularly re-assess pain and other symptoms and implement appropriate interventions promptly • Explore psychosocial impact of pain and other symptoms • Provide high quality care to promote comfort (personal and environmental)	To prevent/effectively manage physical and psychosocial distress
Attachment Aim: to promote caring relationships	• 'Be there' for patient and family when support is needed especially when redefining goals and expectations • Provide a friendly, caring environment which recognises the patient's individuality and needs • Use humour and discussion of 'normal' topics when appropriate • Promote communication and privacy between patients and loved ones to facilitate expressions of caring • Show concern and caring for the family's needs	Demonstrate caring, confirm value and promote some sense of normality Facilitate supportive relationships
Worth Aim: to confirm the patient's value to self and others	• Explore patient's previous experiences and perceptions of illness • Enhance independence utilising appropriate personnel, aids and resources • Explore wishes for future, e.g. desired place of death and promote decision making • Facilitate life review – share personal and family memories • Sensitively explore spiritual/religious beliefs and provide support as appropriate	Affirm worth by respecting individuality, promoting autonomy and respecting beliefs

CASE STUDY 9.4

PARADIGM 1 – FACING IT TOGETHER

Background

Mrs Brown (prefers Ethel) is 75 years old and somewhat frail. Ethel's 76-year-old husband Bill is dying. Although mentally alert, Bill's physical condition is rapidly deteriorating and he is becoming aware of this. The exemplar below was selected as it offers revealing insight into the complex issues inherent in the transition from an awareness context, where staff and relatives collude to conceal the diagnosis from the patient, to a situation of open disclosure.

Ethel: My neighbour had come up to the hospital with me to see my husband. When she asked Bill how he was feeling, he said 'I'd feel a lot better if they'd just tell me the truth. They're all humming and hawing but I know there's something more going on than they're telling me'. Bill was putting two and two together and getting eight. You know what I mean? So I said to him, 'Would you really like to know Bill?' and he said 'Aye, I would. I really would. I'd like to know the truth'.

So I took my neighbour round to the lift and who was coming off the lift but Bill's doctor. The doctor put his arm round my shoulder and he said, 'How are you coping Mrs Brown?' (control slipping – becoming tearful). I said . . . 'Not too bad doctor but the only thing is Bill says he wants to know the truth . . .' The doctor said, 'Well, Mrs Brown if you feel you can tell him then you do that and then I'll come round right behind you'. So I did it. I told Bill, and we both had a wee bubble. Then the doctor came in and he spoke to us both (weeping freely throughout). The doctor was so nice and so gentle. He's a real gentleman . . .

Researcher: How was Bill after you both had your cry together?

Ethel: Well then the doctor came in and I said to him, 'I've told him doctor'. . . . Now he (Bill) just sits and stares into space. When I say to him 'What are you thinking about Bill?', he'll just say, 'Oh everything and nothing'. (silence) Aye. (silence) But I think he'll cope with it all right (sighs).

(Seale 1991, Steptoe et al 1991). Difficulties arising from collusion of this type are poignantly evident in Ethel's account.

In this account, Ethel and Bill's mounting discomfort comes through. As Bill's suspicions grew, he voiced these through the safe medium of a third party (a neighbour), thereby giving Ethel the option either to pick up on his cue or to let it pass.

For Bill, the delicate balance between the pain of knowing, and the distress of *not knowing* had seemingly shifted. Ethel, faced with Bill's question, found further deception impossible. She decided to act on his signal and elected to take on the task of disclosing the grave prognosis to her husband. Ethel's strength and her respect for Bill's 'right to know' stand out.

The doctor came upon Ethel weeping at the lift as she saw her friend off. He responded to her distress and immediately established physical contact and offered comfort. The doctor's suggestion that Ethel should make the disclosure was unusual. Differing views on this decision could usefully be debated. Ethel's judgement was unequivocal: 'The doctor was so nice and so gentle. A real gentleman.' The doctor respected the couple's need for privacy during the disclosure but responded to their subsequent need for support from a caring third party offering to 'come right round and see them both afterwards'.

The enormity of the disclosure had a major impact on Bill. This confirms that even when a patient is seemingly suspicious about their prognosis, denial can operate as a potent defence and hopes of recovery might still be harboured. As Bill absorbed the impact of the news he became quiet and withdrawn and Ethel clearly felt unable to reach him: 'He just sits and stares into space now.' During this part of the interview, Ethel's demeanour was bleak and she was weeping freely.

The interwoven nature of the themes attachment and worth are evident in this extract. The reciprocal character of hope and, indeed, loss of hope were revealed in this account. Ethel's respect for Bill's right to the truth was not without cost. Bill seemed to have slipped away from her. Nevertheless, Ethel seemed hopeful that he would come to terms with what lay ahead. She expressed this as follows: 'Aye, but I think he'll cope with it all right.' The importance of the close attachment of this couple and the capacity for hope to be redirected within a relationship which recognised mutual worth is evident in this case study.

This couple's close relationship had spanned some 52 years and respect for Bill's right to the truth and her own discomfort with the continuing deception led Ethel to act on the cue that her husband had offered. In his seminal study on collusion between spouses, Hinton found that couples caught up in such deception were unable to comfort one another and each partner was left to bear their pain alone (Hinton 1981). Shea and Kendrick confirm this view, suggesting that to face your own death without the benefit of an honest and trusting relationship, could prove an alienating and truly desperate experience (Shea & Kendrick 1995). Ethel and Bill faced it together. (See Reflection point 9B)

Case studies 9.5 and 9.6 offer contrasting examples of relatives' experiences as their loved ones' death drew near. Factors relating to hope and interventions aimed at sustaining hope will be highlighted for discussion.

Comment on Case study 9.5

This Case study emphasises the needs of dying patients and relatives to be in an environment free from intrusive distractions and yet one that offers regular support and attention

---

Reflection point 9B

It is crucial that nurses recognise that for the patient and close family openly to acknowledge the imminence of death can require a shift in emotional orientation within their relationships, of such magnitude, and such profound significance, that for some, it will represent a step quite beyond contemplation. For such families, while there might be tacit acknowledgement of the reality of death, pretence continues to the end. For others, open disclosure of the prognosis is preferred. When this point is reached, hope of recovery is finally dismantled, denial is shelved and the reality of the forthcoming death is confronted openly by the patient and family. In such situations nurses must be acutely sensitive to the needs of the grieving patient and family with all of the implications that this has for their needs for privacy, comfort and support.

---

from staff. By convention, dying patients in hospital tend to be located next to the nurses' station to allow maximum observation and contact. While the logic in this is persuasive, disadvantages were revealed in this account. Sharp insight into the relatives' perspective about the nature of the vigil emerged from these data. An impression emerged of David 'standing

---

CASE STUDY 9.5

PARADIGM 2 – VIGIL DISTURBED

Background

At the time of this interview, David aged 72, was sitting with his wife, Margaret, who sadly died the following day. In his otherwise very positive account David reported the distress which both he and Margaret had experienced as a result of being in the midst of the noise and bustle of a busy surgical ward. Earlier in the interview David had described his discomfort when sitting at his dying wife's bedside in a four-bedded room with several televisions on and other patients' children running around. The data below represent David's response when asked at the end of the interview 'Is there anything else that you would like to add before we finish, David?'.

David: Well . . . I know it's going to sound awful but there was a nurse going down the corridor the other night and the trolley she was pushing was

clattering and squeaking like billy-ho. The door of my wife's room was open because she was feeling claustrophobic . . . (silence)

Researcher: Are you saying that noise . . .

David: Yes. And another thing, the nurses' station is directly opposite Margaret's door. And they keep all the case notes in a trolley right outside her door – and that's where they all congregate to talk. And the ward receptionist has stiletto heels . . . I mean *you* might not hear all that noise going on. But for me. And for Margaret . . . Well you can actually *see* her getting distressed with the noise. Also, the nurses are all nice young lassies but they *do* talk a lot and laugh and giggle a lot. I would like to see the nurses' station with just enough glass up so that the noise is kept inside and with all the files kept in there too. (All said very gently)

Researcher: I see what you mean David. You are in a hub of activity just when you want to be at your most peaceful with Margaret.

within the acute setting as death draws near. Finally, Case study 9.6 (vigil supported) reveals the benefits that relatives can derive from a welcoming and friendly ward environment and from access to facilities for the family's comfort and rest. The hope-sustaining aspects of these interventions are clearly revealed in this account.

McIntyre's work has revealed that threats to hope in relatives may come from a range of sources that include witnessing the deterioration in the condition of their loved one and grief associated with their own impending loss. It confirms that evidence of suffering in the patient results in significant distress in the relative. Difficulties in gaining access to the staff and to information about their loved one's condition causes considerable distress to relatives, robbing them of any sense of control over their situation. Finally, when basic facilities for the comfort and privacy of the visiting family are lacking, stress in relatives is exacerbated.

Of particular interest is the inverse relationship that exists between factors found to generate distress and factors found to foster hope. Furthermore, there is evidence to suggest that as a person's exposure to stress increases either in the intensity or the number of stressors encountered, the capacity of that individual to sustain hope is diminished. It follows from this that the coping resources required to manage stress and the strategies which can be applied to support these coping resources are intricately linked to the capacity of a person to sustain hope.

Nurses can support and sustain hope in relatives, and therefore also in patients, by maintaining a caring presence, by providing for the physical and emotional comfort of the family, by ensuring optimal comfort and care for the dying patient and by offering regular information (Herth 1993, McIntyre 1996). Crucially, staff must establish a sense of their availability to relatives so that supportive relationships can be formed and hopefulness in both patient and the family can be facilitated (Herth 1993, McIntyre 1996).

A HOLISTIC FOCUS FOR HOPE

The research data presented confirm that hope is a complex phenomenon within human experience. The trithematic model used so far in this chapter is useful for the analysis of the concept of hope. It should be stressed that the main themes of comfort, attachment and worth are unique, interwoven and dynamic: each affecting the other. However, while useful for analysis, the model adopted has its limitations as it may fail to fully capture the dynamic and interrelated nature of hope. Furthermore, practitioners are cautioned against adopting too narrow a focus as by doing so they may fail to recognise their potential in supporting hope in those affected by advanced illness.

To address these limitations a symbolic model which seeks to capture and represent the more holistic integrated characteristic of hope is now offered. The dynamic interrelated characteristics of the themes of comfort, attachment and worth within the experience of advanced illness are captured in the image of the butterfly.

The butterfly illustration (see Fig. 9.4) represents a creative attempt to present the key elements of the conceptual model in a visually memorable and symbolic way. The butterfly offers a particularly apt symbol for hope in palliative care. Representing transition and vulnerability, the fragile beauty of the butterfly has the capacity to raise the spirit. Even though its grip on life may be tenuous, the soaring butterfly transcends all that is mundane in a truly spectacular fashion. It is both joyful and poignant. The authors offer the butterfly model as a representation of the hope that is at the heart of palliative nursing care.

It is hoped that the use of a butterfly as a symbol of hope captures some of the features of hope. Its capacity to transcend raises the mood and spirit and generates joyfulness while sharing the fragility and vulnerability of hope. It is an apt symbol for life and hope.

CONCLUSION

This chapter has sought to offer the palliative care nurse an analysis of hope that has utility for practice. Consequently, some of the deeper philosophical explorations of hope have been sacrificed. This was a conscious choice. Readers

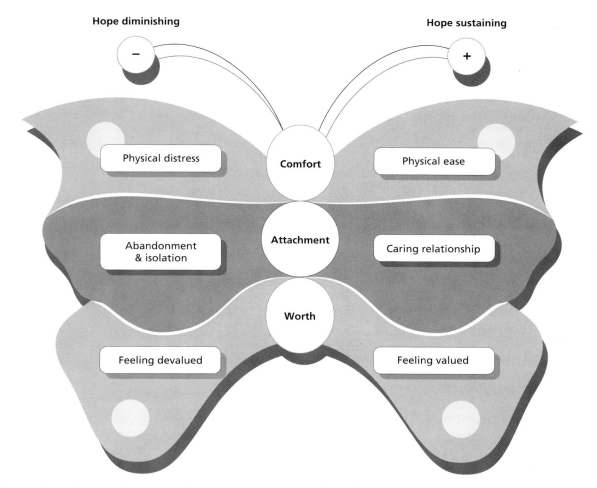

Figure 9.4   The butterfly model of hope: a conceptual model for exploring experiences and interventions.

seeking a deeper analysis of the topic are directed to the growing and diverse body of literature in this field.

The key messages the authors would like to leave with the readers are as follows:

- In essence, hope is about the inner human potential to cope with adversity and to grow as a person. Facilitating hope therefore supports the potential of the individual for self-knowledge and personal growth. However, our current understanding of hope as a concept lacks maturity, especially in the context of palliative care.
- A tri-thematic conceptual model is offered as a useful approach for practising nurses

to help them to explore the concept of hope with patients and relatives and to provide them with a framework from which hope-nurturing strategies can be employed. A word of caution is offered, however; while it may be useful to analyse hope and offer this model for conceptual clarity, humans are integrated holistic beings and holistic care is as fundamental to fostering hope as it is to palliative care. The reciprocal nature of hope demands a family-centred approach to care which encompasses the physical, emotional, social and spiritual.

- Fundamental to the notion of palliative rehabilitation is the belief that it is possible to promote hope and to engender a belief in a better tomorrow even in the profoundly distressing situation of incurable illness.

- The challenge for nurses is to integrate their approaches to fostering hope with their other activities in providing palliative care, e.g. symptom management. This can be difficult. Nurses need to recognise when their problem-solving skills are appropriate, e.g. in symptom management, and when it is more appropriate to employ their facilitative communication skills and simply share the journey with their patients and their relatives.

- Hope is inextricably interwoven with caring. The human spirit is a dynamic force within each person. The energy behind this force needs to be replenished regularly if a sense of hopefulness is to be maintained. Incurable illness has the potential to drain the person of energy, leaving their spirit depleted with the attendant risk of descent into despair and hopelessness.

- High-quality care, therefore, should be focused on restoring the energy in patients and relatives. Promoting physical comfort, confirming the intrinsic worth of the patient and acknowledging the value of family relationships within palliative care are central to hope-directed nursing care.

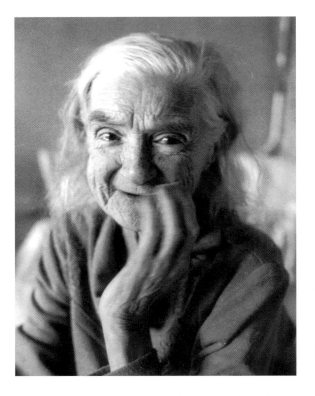

Figure 9.5 Esther: photograph by Colin Dickson from the exhibition 'Remaining Human: Photographs of People with Cancer', reproduced with kind permission of the photographer and the patient/ family.

REFERENCES

Averill J R, Catlin G, Schon K K 1990 Rules of hope. Springer-Verlag, New York
Byock I 1996 Beyond symptom management. European Journal of Palliative Care 3(3): 125–130
Carse J P 1980 Death and existence. Wiley, New York
Chaplin J 1996 An exploration of the quality of care received by individuals having lung cancer surgery: perceptions of patients, relatives and nurses. Dissertation, University of Glasgow
de Raeve L 1996 Dignity and integrity at the end of life. International Journal of Palliative Nursing 2(2): 71–76
Dufault K, Martocchio B 1985 Hope: its spheres and dimensions. Nursing Clinics of North America 20(2): 379–391
Farrer A 1992 How much do they want to know? Communicating with dying patients. Professional Nurse 7(9): 606–609
Flemming K 1997 The meaning of hope to palliative care cancer patients. International Journal of Palliative Nursing 3(1): 14–18

Glaser B, Strauss A 1965 Awareness of dying. Aldine, Chicago
Herth K A 1990 Fostering hope in terminally ill people. Journal of Advanced Nursing 15: 1250–1259
Herth K A 1993 Hope in the family caregiver of terminally ill people. Journal of Advanced Nursing 18: 538–548
Hinton J 1981 Sharing or withholding information of dying between husband and wife. Journal of Psychosomatic Research 25: 337–343
Hockley J 1993 The concept of hope and the will to live. Palliative Medicine 7: 181–186
Hodson P 1990 Whose death is it anyway? The Observer, 11 March 1990. Cited in Hunt G 1991 The truth about terminal cancer. Nursing 4(40): 9–11
Hull M M 1989 Family needs and supportive nursing behaviours during terminal cancer. A review. Oncology Nursing Forum 16(6): 787–792
Hunt M 1991 The truth about terminal cancer. Nursing (Oxford) 4(40): 9–11
Kubler-Ross E 1969 On death and dying. Macmillan, New York

Lair G S 1996 Counselling the terminally ill. Taylor & Francis Ltd, Washington

Lazarus R S 1993 Coping theory and research: past, present, and future. Psychosomatic Medicine 55: 234–247

Maslow A 1968 Towards a psychology of being. Van Nostrand Reinhold, New York

McIntyre R 1996 Nursing support for relatives of dying cancer patients in hospital: Improving standards by research. Doctoral Thesis, Glasgow Caledonian University

McIntyre R 1991 Support for family and carers. In: Lugton J, Kindlen M (eds) Palliative care: the nursing role. Churchill Livingstone, Edinburgh, pp. 193–215

Nugent L S 1998 The social support requirements of family caregivers of terminal cancer patients. Canadian Journal of Nursing Research 20(3): 45–58

Pearlin L, Schooler C 1978 The structure of coping. Journal of Health and Social Behaviour 19(March): 2–21

Perakyla A 1991 Hope work in the care of seriously ill patients. Qualitative Health Research 1(4): 407–433

Post-White J, Ceronsky C, Kreitzer M J et al 1996 Hope, spirituality, sense of coherence, and quality of life in patients with cancer. Oncology Nursing Forum 23(10): 1571–1578

Rogers C 1961 On becoming a person. Houghtlin-Mifflin, Boston

Russell G 1993 The role of denial in clinical practice. Journal of Advanced Nursing 18(6): 938–940

Saunders C 1984 The management of terminal illness. Edward Arnold, London

Scanlon C 1989 Creating a vision of hope: the challenge of palliative care. Oncology Nursing Forum 16(4): 491–496

Seale C 1991 Communicating and awareness about death – a study of a random sample of dying people. Social Science & Medicine 32(8): 943–952

Shea T, Kendrick K 1995 With velvet gloves: the ethics of collusion. Palliative Care Today 4(1): 9–10

Steptoe A, Sutcliffe I, Allen B, Coombes C 1991 Satisfaction with communication, medical knowledge, and coping style in patients with metastatic cancer. Social Science and Medicine 32(6): 627–632

10

Bereavement, grief and mourning

Sally Anstey   Mel Lewis

Anything that you have, you can lose,
Anything you are attached to, you can be separated
  from;
Anything you love can be taken away from you,
Yet, if you really have nothing to lose, you have
  nothing.

(Kalish 1985)

This chapter is concerned with bereavement, grief and mourning in adult life. It seeks to explore the ways people experience grief and how others impact on this experience within the context of Western society. It will concentrate on exploring these issues in relation to palliative care.

As you read this chapter consider the fact that just over a quarter of the adult population will be experiencing the death of someone close, who has died within the last 5 years (Littlewood 1992). For some that death will be sudden and unexpected; for others it will be as the result of a long illness and expected. It may be that this death is the first to be encountered by the bereaved individual or it may be one of many bereavements already experienced.

The impact and effect of the bereavement, however, is an individual response and can span the whole spectrum of human emotions.

Despite often being associated with traumatic events, bereavement, grief and mourning are all inherent throughout our lives, linking closely to aspects of change. Our individual and societal attitudes towards dying and bereavement are not innate: our culture and our responses to life experience, both personal and professional, shape them.

It is also important to acknowledge that early in the 21st century the way we approach living and ageing has a direct relationship on the way we die and grieve.

THEORETICAL BACKGROUND

The dominant theories and models associated with bereavement that have emerged in the 20th century have been derived from psychological and sociological thinking which supports the process of adjustment following a structured process of separation from the dead person; this has been described as 'grief work'.

Think:

- Freud
- Lindemann
- Bowlby

New models and thoughts are evolving which challenge the 'grief work' assumption of 'dealing with' the past before moving on. They consider the importance of the 'continuing presence' of the dead person in the life of the bereaved as being essential in 'defining their past and shaping their future'. This is a very new concept, but challenges us to reconsider our approach to bereaved individuals.

The key proponents of this are:

- Walter
- Stroebe

The rationale behind many of the theoretical frameworks developed is to provide a guide for professionals in understanding and supporting people with their losses and throughout the bereavement trajectory.

Bereavement, grief and mourning

It is important to explore what we understand by bereavement, grief and mourning. There are definitions that suggest a link between loss of something precious and the consequent emotional and psychological responses.

Wendell-Moller (1996) clarifies the definitions as follows:

- 'Bereavement is an essential component of grief. Literally speaking, to be bereaved means to be deprived, to have something taken away. . . . Bereavement can be defined as the sense of deprivation or loss generated by the loss of another person.'
- 'Grief is an intense emotional response to bereavement that involves sorrow and suffering . . . bereavement precedes grief but is not necessarily followed by it.'
- 'Mourning is the behavioural and ritualistic expression of the emotional anguish of grief but may not always reflect inner feelings.'

From the above definitions it is apparent that there is both linkage and overlap between bereavement, grief and mourning but also that these are clear distinctions.

Reflection point

- Death is an almost universal experience.
- We will all lose through death:
  - family members
  - friends
  - peers
  - colleagues.
- This death will be marked by:
  - emotional responses → *Grief*
  - behavioural rituals → *Mourning*.
- Death involves personal and private, individual and social manifestations, which are culturally and socially established.
- The impact of bereavement is unique to the individual and there is no 'prescription' to guide the professional role.

Models and theories of grief have been developed to help us more clearly understand and support people who have been bereaved. The following section describes, categorises and critically appraises some of the more familiar models and theories of grief, putting them into an historical and cultural context and exploring their usefulness in the clinical setting with particular emphasis on palliative care. The words 'models' and 'theories' are often used interchangeably – they are not the same but are complementary to each other (Box 10.1).

> **Box 10.1**   Models and theories
>
> A *model* describes both what happens when someone is grieving and how the experience impacts on the person and their life whereas a *theory* tries to explain both what happens when someone is grieving, and why he or she experiences it in the way they do – cause and effect (Parkes 1998).

Phase models of grief

Key points

- Derived from the work of Bowlby, who explored the attachment bonds between mother and child, which are instinctive and important for survival, and suggested that damage to these bonds in early life directly influences the security or insecurity of future relationships.
- He categorised the reactions of children when separated from their mother into three phases:

  1. angry pining
  2. depression and despair
  3. detachment.

- This was adapted and applied to bereaved adults in the 1970s by Bowlby and Parkes who, following extensive research, added a new first phase of *numbness*.
- Elizabeth Kubler-Ross (1969) has applied this phase approach to individuals' psychological adaptation to the diagnosis of life-threatening illness.

Strengths

- Described empirically and attempted a classification of the process of grieving.
- Recognised that it was not possible to develop a 'prescription' for grieving.
- Acknowledged the 'roller coaster' nature of the emotions/behaviours associated with grief and mourning.
- First postulated the idea of transitions that have subsequently become an important concept in palliative care.

Weaknesses

- They have been misused by some as a prescription or template for grieving – ignoring the individuality of the experience.
- Do not fully acknowledge the cultural and ethnic variation in the expression of grief.

Relevance to practice

- It offers a helpful hint when undertaking family assessments to explore their responses to past losses, as they may be a guide to predict or understand current responses.
- New research indicates that attachment theory may be predictive of complicated grieving – if this is proven it may help us determine 'at risk' individuals and link them to specialist services.
- Marrone (1997) cited by Clark & Seymour (1999) gives an in-depth analysis of eight different phase theories that have evolved from Bowlby's work.

The medical model of grief

Key points

- Derived from the work of Lindemann (1944) at the end of the Second World War.
- Demonstrates that grief is a sickness, similar to a disease.
- As a disease it indicates that grief displays symptoms, e.g. pain and disturbed physical/mental functions.
- Suggests that grief is a physiological stress and also contributes to the manifestation of symptoms, both physical and psychological.
- Indicates that for some individuals grieving is 'abnormal' and by implication suggests that the 'bereaved person is sick or mentally ill'.

Strengths

- Indicates and acknowledges that overt physical and psychological symptoms are a 'normal' consequence of bereavement.
- Defining someone as ill may entitle them to certain benefits, e.g. access to treatments, but

conversely may stigmatise them and impact on their role in society.

Weaknesses

- Slightly old research that has largely been superseded.
- It has been viewed, by recent authors, as offensive to categorise some people who are grieving as being mentally ill.
- Ignores societal and cultural differences in the manifestation of grieving and mourning.

Relevance to practice

- Recent research suggests that there are a very small minority of people who experience 'complicated' grieving.
- Suggests that, in practice, we should be more cautious in our categorisation of individuals experiencing grieving difficulties.
- By more appropriate categorisation, the minority of individuals needing the support of mental health professionals might perhaps have easier access.

The grief work model

Key points

- It is a descriptive model, initially identified by Freud (1917), which describes the hard work, time and pain involved in working through grief.
- Links closely to his theory of repression, suggesting that because of the pain involved, people avoid dealing with their loss and attempt to 'hide' their thoughts, feelings and emotions.
- Emphasised the importance of grieving openly, especially in the first few weeks.
- Demonstrated that grieving and mourning were a struggle and necessitated activity similar to that of a job.
- A number of authors have provided evidence to support the view that repression of emotions at the time of death may lead to problems at a later date. (Other authors

suggest that it is the hiding of emotions at any time during grieving that is important, with no particular significance attached to the time of death.)

Strengths

- Acknowledges that grief necessitates hard work.
- Laid the foundations for subsequent theorists' 'stages of responses' (Kubler-Ross 1969) and 'tasks of mourning' (Worden 1991) which identify how the hard work involved can be structured.
- Indicates that emotions should not be hidden and that displaying them may be helpful.

Weaknesses

- Does not acknowledge the difficulties for some individuals in openly showing their emotions.
- It is simplistic to assume that emotional repression is the only cause of complicated grief.
- Does not consider cultural variations in the expression of grief or how the place or manner of the death may influence emotional release.

Relevance to practice

- Indicates the importance of giving the bereaved the time and privacy for emotional release at the time of death; obviously whether people are openly emotional is individually determined – people should not be forced to cry or be emotional if they choose otherwise.
- As professionals we should attempt to feel comfortable with people who are displaying emotions at the time of death, especially if those emotions/behaviours are unusual to us: for example, overt anger/screaming is sometimes more difficult for us to cope with than crying.
- Remember there is marked cultural variation in the expressions of grief and mourning.

Summary

As can be seen the traditional models of bereavement rely on the need for hard work and going through a progression of issues, including acceptance of the loss and continuation of life without the deceased. It ignores the fact that the loss does not occur in isolation and that there are additional factors adding to the impact of the bereavement, and the individual experiences of grief and mourning.

Newer approaches consider a more holistic approach to loss and could perhaps be compared to Saunders' (1978) 'concept of total pain' which contextualises the pain experience. A framework of 'total loss' could include the following components of the individual:

- personal/individual
- physical
- psychological/emotional
- social/cultural
- occupational
- spiritual
- financial

and link it to experience of bereavement, grief and mourning. This framework demonstrates the beginnings of new approaches being explored by Walter (1996) and Stroebe (1998).

Grief, bereavement, biography – a new model

Walter (1996) describes 'a new model of grief: bereavement and biography' as being relevant for a more secular independent society.

Key points

- Opposes/contradicts the view of earlier theorists that concentrates on adaptation to and recovery from grief and ignores its individuality and complexity.
- The aim is to 'reconstruct' the story of the bereaved's relationship with the dead person by sharing their thoughts and feelings with others who have known the dead person.
- The suggested outcome is two-fold:
  i) the strengthening of the attachment to the person who had died
  ii) with the consequence being that it gives meaning and continuity to the life of the survivors.
- Links to earlier work that suggests that many of the bereaved maintain 'spiritual' contact with the person who has died – that it is a common experience. Many bereaved people are frightened to describe this type of experience to others for fear of being 'labelled' as abnormal.

Strengths

- Enables the unique experience to be explored and reflections made linking the past and present in shaping the future of the bereaved.
- Allows for a holistic, multicultural approach, which supports the linkage of life and death in a variety of ways without the use of structured frameworks.
- Encourages individual interpretation of what has happened.

Weaknesses

- Assumes that all bereaved people have someone with whom to share their recollections of the dead person.
- Certain circumstances surrounding their death will render this approach unworkable or more complicated; for example, neonatal death or suicide.
- Relies on conversation and the skills of being able to articulate thoughts, feelings and emotions.
- May encourage one survivor to dominate or shape the responses of others.

Relevance to practice

- Potentially useful in palliative care; links to the concept of anticipatory grief, where there

is time while the person is still alive to fill/clarify some of the gaps in the story.
- Less useful, as an approach, at the time of the death.
- Suggests the benefits of someone who knew the deceased being involved in the support of the survivors facilitates some sharing in the storytelling – this has implications for bereavement services and support programmes.
- Raises our awareness of some of the contextual and personal issues surrounding loss, having direct relevance to us as human beings who are also the potentially bereaved.

The dual process model

Stroebe's more recent work (1996/1998) explored gender differences in coping with loss. As a consequence she developed a model (Fig. 10.1) that she describes as 'a healthy mix of both male and female ways of coping, a confrontation and avoidance of both emotions and problems, an oscillation in attention to these dimensions' (Stroebe 1998, p. 10).

Key points

- Describes loss- versus restoration-orientation.
- Loss-orientation considers the issues in dealing with the bereavement itself; linking closely to the earlier theories of 'grief responses' and 'grief work', this is familiar territory.
- Restoration-orientation is the less well known or acknowledged element which explores the adjustment to changes that occur as a direct result of the loss, but are secondary factors that add to the burden (e.g. dealing with the finances or cooking).
- The model relies on the idea of 'oscillation' – that there is active movement of the individual between issues associated with the loss or with restoration.
- It also suggests that individuals cope with the experience by continually moving from confrontation and acceptance to denial and distraction.

Strengths

- Places the individual's experience of bereavement in the 'real world' as part of life and not separate from it.

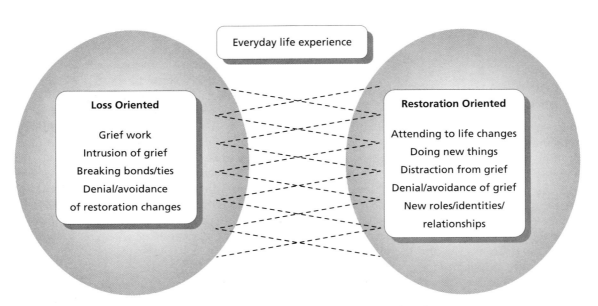

Figure 10.1 A dual process model of coping with loss, adapted from Stroebe (1998).

- Makes understandable both the 'roller-coaster' nature of the experience of bereavement and the responses to it. Clearly links to adaptation theories and transitions (as discussed in Chapter 7).
- Has been developed supported by pictorial representation, which aids understanding.

Weaknesses

- Relies on men and women being able to move between their relative 'comfort zones' in adjusting to bereavement.
- Identifies prescriptively that men are more comfortable in dealing with the practical issues and women are more able to confront the emotions involved – research supports this but there are likely to be a small number of individuals not so easily categorised.
- The approach has not been validated/ explored beyond the Western-Caucasian cultures so its relevance to other cultures would benefit from exploration. (Stroebe herself suggests this is a limitation.)
- Are these gender differences relevant in promoting our understanding of same-sex partner bereavement?

Relevance to practice

- By increasing our awareness of gender differences in coping we may be able to develop more appropriate supportive frameworks.
- In palliative care, as part of anticipatory grief work, it might be possible to consider the potential additional stresses (e.g. cooking or money management) and develop approaches for passing on these skills either from the dying person themselves or from appropriate support services.
- When working with families it may be helpful to explore the issues of gender differences and how it impacts on individuals coping. It may increase understanding and tolerance of the manifest differences.

- It will help us as people and professionals to understand more about the 'normal' experiences associated with grief and mourning and to be more appropriately supportive.

The authors consider it important to include a critical appraisal of anticipatory grief; it is a theoretical concept that may be useful when considering the bereavement trajectory.

Anticipatory grief

Key points

- It is a concept, initially identified by Lindemann (1944), that describes grief and mourning that occurs in anticipation of the death event.
- It has been used to explore and explain some of the emotional and behavioural reactions of patients with cancer and their families/ friends.
- The evidence from the literature is mixed as to whether anticipatory grieving exists or whether undertaking grief work with patients and families before the death is useful.

Strengths

- It provides a useful framework to understand and explore the reactions and behaviours of patients with cancer and their families.
- Evidence suggests that anticipatory grief work allows for emotional and practical adjustments to be made which may modify the impact of the death for the bereaved.

Weaknesses

- Its relevance and existence remains open to debate – the boundaries are blurred with spiritual and psychological distress.
- It may help the bereaved at the expense of the dying person (this may also be a strength).
- Its long-term benefit in impacting on bereavement outcome is uncertain.

Relevance to practice

- Useful for people with advanced cancer and their families who cope with stressful events by planning, discussing and exploring all the issues associated with the death. (There may be dissonance within families.)
- Requires professionals to be equally open in their communication and information giving.
- Its use for people dying from other life-threatening illnesses, where the dying trajectory is less predictable and often more protracted, may be troublesome (Lewis 1996).

Conclusion

Explaining bereavement, grief and mourning in theoretical terms is both helpful and problematic: *helpful* in that it gives us a number of possible explanations for a person's experience; *problematic* in that 'theories' implies a progression from cause and effect to management and resolution.

The describing of a number of theories models in this chapter is to enable you to consider a variety of approaches in your support of the bereaved.

THE LINK BETWEEN THEORY AND PRACTICE

A Buddhist legend tells the story of bereavement, grief and mourning that both attempts to describe the cause, effect and outcomes of the experience, but rightly puts the person at the centre of the situation:

In India, a woman called Kisa-Gotami whose son had died went around her village with the dead child in her arms looking for a cure. People thought she was crazy.

She went to see the Buddha and asked him to give her some medicine to cure her son. The Buddha realised that she had not encountered death before. He said he would help, if she would come back to him bringing a mustard seed from every household where no one had died.

Following her journey she failed to bring back a single mustard seed but in the process learnt that death was universal, that she was not the only

mother whose child had died and was finally able to let him go.   (Parkes 1998)

> **Reflection point**
>
> How does this link with your reading related to the theoretical background of bereavement, grief and mourning?
>   Have you considered:
>
> - the phases of grief
> - gender/cultural differences
> - the 'work' involved in grieving and mourning
> - biography or lack of it

BEREAVEMENT: EXPERIENCES OF GRIEF

Before moving on to consider the individual experience of grief, it is important to consider the more universal experiences and attempt to categorise the thoughts, feelings and behaviours of the bereaved (Fig. 10.2).

The emotions experienced by the bereaved fluctuate over time; they can be apparent before the death and can continue for a number of years after the death (Fig. 10.3).

Early authors indicate the emotions take many years to resolve (Gorer 1965), whereas Smith (1982) predicted that the experience should be less intense after 6 months. Parkes (1972) indicated that grief might be problematic if it lasts over a year.

This, however, fails to acknowledge the additional stresses faced by the bereaved such as the lifestyle change that impacts on the grieving process (Holmes & Rahe 1967). Some authors (see previous paragraph) have attempted to estimate the time taken to 'recover' or 'adapt' to bereavement. The evidence remains equivocal.

Time limits are often unhelpful; they are not a valid outcome measure determining successful adjustment. Timeliness of the bereaved person's emotional responses may be helpful in:

- further understanding the experience of uncomplicated grief

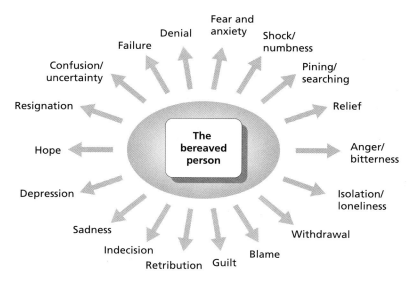

Figure 10.2 Possible emotions experienced by the bereaved. (Adapted from work developed by Stroebe & Stroebe 1987, Littlewood 1992, Penson & Fisher 1995, and others.)

• hinting at/predicting possible difficulties.

Additional physical responses commonly reported by bereaved people are as follows (adapted from Worden 1991, cited by Littlewood 1992):

• experience of hollowness associated with the stomach or abdomen
• experience of tightness, especially in the chest/throat/shoulders
• increased sensitivity/awareness of noise
• breathlessness/deep sighing respirations
• muscle weakness
• fatigue and lack of energy
• dry mouth and increased effort in swallowing.

Being aware of the physical sensations and behavioural responses associated with loss enables us to support the already vulnerable bereaved and explain that although these experiences are fearful, they are rarely cause for concern. Additionally, in palliative care, the person may display symptoms similar to those experienced by the deceased. This may be problematic, as they may be convinced that they are suffering from the same disease. Despite their normality, these symptoms and sensations need to be explored and the timing of their emergence fol-

lowing the bereavement needs to be elicited to exclude any possible pathological cause or need for active interventions (see Grief counselling – Level 3, later).

Remember

There is much research evidence linking the death of a loved person with increased mortality and morbidity for the survivors, especially within the first 6 months of the bereavement (Young et al 1963, Parkes 1972, Kalish 1985, Worden 1991). Most, but not all, of this evidence is derived from work on spousal bereavement but it can be applied to other types of partner loss.

FACTORS IMPACTING ON THE INDIVIDUAL EXPERIENCE OF LOSS

In practice, it is clear that there are other issues to consider when exploring the impact of bereavement, grief and mourning. These factors may positively or negatively impact on the individual's experience.

When supporting family members around the time of death, consider:

1. The nature of the bereaved person's relationship with the deceased: e.g.

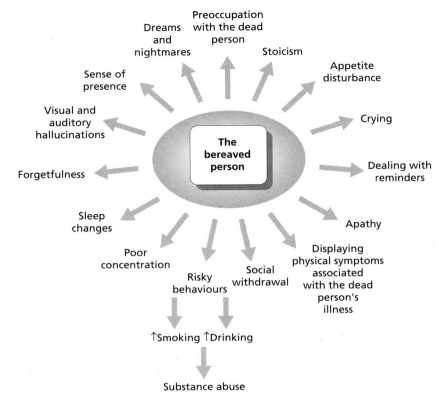

Figure 10.3 Possible behavioural and physical responses experienced by the bereaved (not an exhaustive list).

ambivalent (Raphael 1984), dependent (Parkes 1972).

2. The manner and the timing of the death:
   - when the bereaved are not present (Worden 1991)
   - when an unpleasant event happens at the time of death.
3. Whether the death was expected or unexpected:
   - unanticipated/sudden (Parkes 1972)
   - as a result of suicide/self-neglect (Kalish 1985).
4. The age of the person who dies:
   - A child at whatever age! If it is a young child or an adult child with elderly parents it may be seen as an 'untimely death' (Worden 1991, Young & Cullen 1996).
5. The perceived 'social worth' of the dead person within the social scene:

- shameful life or shameful death (Lazare 1979, cited by Littlewood 1992)
- poor social support networks (Vachon et al 1982, cited by Littlewood 1992).

Reflection point

How do the above link to preparing families/ friends for a person's death from life-threatening illness?

There is no 'foolproof' way of determining exactly which bereavements will have either an overwhelming or transitory impact on the survivors and their future life:

- Think of Queen Victoria!

For her, the death of her husband was a personal event but because of her position it was open to public scrutiny and led to much professional interest in bereavement:

- it was a highly dependent relationship
- she was not present at the time of death
- the death was sudden
- Prince Albert was relatively young
- as a Queen, her social support system may have been depersonalised due to her perceived and actual status.

Depending on your age or your memory:

- Think of the Aberfan Disaster in the early 1960s.
- Think of the Hillsborough Disaster in the late 1980s.
- Think of the death of Diana, Princess of Wales in 1997.
- Think of the Paddington Train Crash in 1999.

British people are described as being reserved and likely to conceal their emotions. Historically, traditional rituals following death provided a framework to enable us to openly grieve and express distress. These traditions weakened, largely as a response to societal change and increasing secularisation, and the bereaved are confused by current expectation that values emotional reserve and stifles public displays of grief. This changed with the death of the Princess of Wales in 1997, but confusion is still perpetuated by the debate as to which is the healthier way of expressing grief: repression or expression. Walter (1997) contends that expressing grief openly is natural and its repression is harmful, but suggests that public behaviour is governed by social rules, which leaves many people uncertain as to how to grieve and behave. This situation is additionally complicated by the influence of the media, which has made intensely private and personal bereavements part of the public domain.

It is uncertain how the media influences the private experiences of bereavement and grief. It is generally acknowledged that the media may either 'prescribe' certain responses or 'desensitise' individuals as to their own feelings and as a consequence manipulate their responses. It is possible that a similar manifestation was apparent at the time of 'Live Aid'; commentators recognised the concept of 'famine fatigue', where people ceased to be disturbed by intensely distressing sights of starvation and deprivation.

Thus, it is clear that the media has some responsibility in influencing grief, and this is unlikely to lessen in the future. The major concern is related to its mixed message – whereby violent death is commonplace on our screens, but a 'natural death' due to be screened in winter 1998 was almost barred from television by court injunction.

Many authors accept that the thoughts, feelings, emotions and behaviours that are manifest as a consequence of bereavement are 'socially determined'; they are further mediated by the historical and cultural context of the society in which the death occurs (this has been alluded to earlier in the chapter).

THEORY → PRACTICE: PROBLEM-SOLVING IN PALLIATIVE CARE

This chapter has so far concentrated on the theoretical background that supports discussion surrounding bereavement, grief and mourning. It has described both research and anecdotal studies, but does any of this help us in dealing with problems and issues in palliative care practice?

The care and support we as professionals are able to offer the bereaved individual is related to three key factors:

1. The care setting in which the death occurred.
2. The stage of the grieving trajectory where the individual is 'at'.
3. The knowledge, skills and comfort we as individuals (despite our professional role) feel in relation to our care of the bereaved.

A straw poll of colleagues has indicated that for most professionals bereavement texts seem to be strong on the theoretical background but less helpful in describing strategies to help those grieving. This may be appropriate, as it is

Intermediate/specialist bereavement – care is provided by specialist practitioners usually working in non-specialist settings/areas or those not exclusively working in a counselling role.

Level 2 interventions related to the specialist providing 'direct care' may include:

- A bereavement problem has been identified either by the generalist health/social care team or by lay carers or the bereaved person.
- A holistic assessment is facilitated or undertaken by the appropriate specialist using a validated tool or evidence-based approach.
- A strategy is developed to deal with any particular problem or to facilitate normal grieving.
- The interventions are undertaken either by:
  (i) the referrer with support and guidance
  (ii) the appropriate specialist within an agreed timescale and providing demonstrable outcomes.

Level 2 'indirect care' is very similar to 'direct care'. The distinctions relate to the consultative role of the specialist practitioner or service:

- They provide a specialist resource related to bereavement care.
- As part of their role they encourage discussion of the particular experience of death and offer support as appropriate to lay or professional carers, but *not* to the bereaved person.
- They facilitate and educate health and social care professionals in the use of tools/evidence to assess and/or manage those at risk from complicated grief.

Level 3: Complex/specialist bereavement – counselling

The strategies appropriate to this level are those developed by advanced level practitioners or specialist services with expertise in one or more of the following areas: clinical psychology, counselling, family therapy or social work. This expertise is developed and validated by being used consistently in a professional or therapeutic arena (NCHSPCS 2000).

The different disciplines acknowledged as demonstrating this expertise include psychiatrists, clinical psychologists, counsellors, social workers, family therapists and spiritual advisers. The aim of level 3 interventions is to employ: 'Those specialised techniques . . . which are used to help people with abnormal or complicated grief reactions' (Worden 1991). The specialised techniques may include, but not exclusively, psychotherapy, counselling, behavioural and cognitive therapies.

These interventions provide specialist grief counselling to the minority of people experiencing abnormal or complicated grief reactions. Complicated grief (also described as abnormal or pathological grief) has been described as:

a *deviation* from the normal, expected grieving reaction that relates to the particular bereavement the individual experienced.   (Littlewood 1992)

Deviation may be related to:

- The *duration* of the grieving reaction = Chronic grief
- The *inhibition* of the specific/general symptoms of grief which become more intense with subsequent losses = Delayed grief
- The *overwhelming* nature of the grief which may lead to addictive or depressive behaviours = Exaggerated grief

The most common deviation is usually related to the duration of grieving.

For most professionals the complexity and depth of skills required to facilitate complicated grief are not part of their day-to-day work. Their responsibility is to identify these reactions and negotiate referral to more specialist services. (This section acknowledges the National Hospice Council's publications related to psychosocial care.)

Using the levels of intervention in relation to bereavement may have the following advantages:

- The bereaved individual experiencing the 'roller-coaster' nature of grieving may need professionals who are alert to the changes and able to respond and refer on appropriately.
- It provides a developmental framework for professionals in relation to skills acquisition and may enable the identification of competencies for practice.
- Supports practitioners in admitting that they do not have or do not necessarily need all of the answers. It facilitates them in using other professionals/agencies to support their care.
- It acknowledges the importance of considering the ethical impact of our care. In particular, the principles of beneficence and non-maleficence, 'to do good' and 'to do no harm', by our interventions. Anecdotally, some bereaved individuals have been harmed by professional 'dabbling' that is not supported by appropriate knowledge/skills.
- It will support the development of standards of care for individual services and relevant outcome measures.

Reflection point

From these identified advantages a major criticism of this approach may lie in its concentration on the professional role to the marginalisation of the individual person's experience of bereavement: What do you think?

Practical considerations

There are difficulties in supporting individualised care for the bereaved. The following are specific areas worthy of attention (see Case study 10.1).

Risk identification

Awareness of risk factors impacting on bereavement outcome is important in prioritising the activity of specialist services. However, authors do not agree either as to what is a risk factor or how to weight the identified risks (Osterweiss et al 1984). Faull et al (1998, p. 83) provide a useful list:

CASE STUDY 10.1

Maggie, 58 years old, has been admitted with end-stage breast cancer. Her disease was diagnosed as metastatic one year ago. Since her admission in the early hours of the morning her condition has deteriorated; Maggie has been semi-conscious for the last 2 hours and she is clearly dying.

Her husband, William, has been with her throughout the night and is clearly distraught. He appears alone and isolated and clearly appears desperate to talk to someone. He admits that he has not talked to his daughters from his first marriage about Maggie having breast cancer for fear of distressing them as their mother died of breast cancer aged 39 years.

William has become more tearful and distraught and states that he must be to blame in some way for what has happened because how could this happen twice? He becomes more distressed when you mention contacting his daughters.

It is apparent that William has both actual and potential needs.

With your knowledge of bereavement what particular issues and risk factors do you identify in relation to William's story?

What level of intervention do you assess William requires and why?

How will you either deliver that intervention or action other professionals to achieve the required intervention?

What measures would help you identify that William's needs are being met?

Reflection points
Consider links to the main section of the chapter:

- Theories/Models
- Feelings/Emotions/Behaviours
- Levels of bereavement intervention

- younger age (of the deceased)
- poor social support
- sudden death
- previous poor physical and mental health
- limited coping strategies
- multiple losses/unresolved grief
- stigmatised death
- financial difficulties.

Useful additions to the list could be:

- personality variables (Vachon et al 1982)
- people with learning disabilities (Kitching 1987).

It perhaps is useful to consider the risk factors as a useful checklist. The relative importance of each may change over time and may be influenced by the impact of the particular loss.

Family variables

It is crucial to consider each family member as an individual. Their individual risk factors, coping strategies and bereavement responses are likely to be unique and linked to their relationship with the deceased (spouse, partner, parent, sibling, child, friend, colleague, lover). The family unit as a whole may influence whether individuals cope with the loss positively or negatively.

Transitions

The impact of the bereavement and the needs of the bereaved may change over time. External events may impact on the bereavement experience; for individuals, changes in their role and responsibilities may complicate adaptation.

The 4 Rs

It is important to match the individual needing bereavement intervention to the:
• *Right* provider
• At the *Right* time
• Using the *Right* approach
• To achieve the *Right* outcomes.

In this context, *Right* = Right for the individual.
It is important for all professionals to ensure that referral policies and protocols are in place to support seamless and speedy access to specialists and bereavement services. In consultation with the bereaved individual this should be implemented when 'staff recognise they have reached the ceiling of their skills, or (when) the situation has become too complex' (NCHSPCS 1993). (See also useful organisations in the Appendix to this chapter.)

Evidence

There is limited published evidence that demonstrates any evaluation as to the effectiveness of bereavement interventions. Of the variety of strategies employed, none have been evaluated. In developing a framework for bereavement care, it is important to consider the quality initiative of clinical governance (Lugon & Secker-Walker 1999). Some of the core elements may provide a useful guide to identify appropriate

care of the bereaved throughout the grieving trajectory, the most relevant, perhaps, being:

• risk management
• evidence-based practice
• standards
• audit
• peer review
• ongoing professional development
• management of poor performance
• clinical supervision
• multi-professional working
• patient and carer satisfaction.

Reflection point

Consider how bereavement care is organised in your clinical setting.

• What changes might make it more appropriate for the bereaved?
• What changes might make it more appropriate for the multi-professional team?
• How compatible are these changes?

CONCLUSION

The subject of grief, bereavement and mourning is vast, complex and challenging. As human beings both in our personal and professional lives we will experience bereavement and our responses will be individual. As nurses, we have the responsibility to support individuals experiencing the variety of bereavement responses, but the accountability to ensure that we recognise our own limitations and access specialist help appropriately.

ACKNOWLEDGEMENTS

The authors would like to acknowledge the work of the many professional colleagues who postulated and developed the concepts of levels of care and intervention (especially Jeanette Webber, Ilora Finlay and Peter Tebbit) and to Professor David Field's Briefing paper No. 4 (2000) which provided a 'Eureka' moment! Thanks also to the Editors for their patience and to Val Williams for her extraordinary computer skills.

REFERENCES

Bowling A, Cartwright A 1982 Life after death: study of elderly widows. Tavistock, London

Clark D, Seymour J 1999 Reflections on palliative care. Open University Press, Buckingham

Concise Oxford English Dictionary 1990 8th edn. Clarendon Press, Oxford

Davies B, Reimer J K, Brown P, Martens N 1995 Fading away. The experience of transition in families with terminal illness. Baywood Publishing Company Inc., New York

Davis B D, Cowley S A, Ryland R K 1996 The effects of terminal illness on patients and their carers. Journal of Advanced Nursing 23: 512–520

Faull C, Carter Y, Woof R (eds) 1998 Handbook of palliative care. Blackwell, Oxford

Freihofer P, Felton G 1976 Nursing behaviours in bereavement: an exploratory study. Nursing Research 25: 332–337

Freud S 1917 Morning and melancholic. In: Standard Edition of the Complete Psychological Works of Sigmund Freud, Vol. 14. Hogarth Press, London

Gorer I 1965 Death, grief and mourning in contemporary Britain. Doubleday, New York

Hampe S O 1975 The needs of grieving spouses in a hospital setting. Nursing Research 24: 113–119

Holmes T H, Rahe R H 1967 The social readjustment rating scale. Journal of Psychosomatic Research 2: 213–218

Hull M M 1989 Family needs and supporting nursing behaviours during terminal cancer, a review. Oncology Nursing Forum 16: 787–792

Kalish R A 1985 Death, grief and caring relationships, 2nd edn. Brooks Cole, California

Kitching N 1987 Helping people with mental handicap: a case study with discussion. Journal of the British Institute of Mental Handicap 15: 60–63

Kubler-Ross E 1969 On death and dying. Tavistock, London

Lewis M A 1996 Anticipatory grief. Unpublished dissertation, University of Wales College of Medicine

Lindemann E 1944 Symptomatology and the management of acute grief. American Journal of Psychiatry 101 (September): 141–148

Littlewood J 1992 Aspects of grief: bereavement in adult life. Routledge, London

Lugon M, Secker-Walker J 1999 Clinical governance making it happen. Royal Society of Medicine Press Limited, UK/USA

National Council for Hospice and Specialist Palliative Care Services (NCHSPCS) 1993 In: Higginson I (ed.) Matching services to individual needs. NCHSPC, London

National Council for Hospice and Specialist Palliative Care Services (NCHSPCS) 1999 Palliative Care 2000: Commissioning palliative care services. NCHSPC, London

National Council for Hospice and Specialist Palliative Care Services (NCHSPCS) 2000 Briefing No. 4: What do we mean by 'Psychosocial' (written by D. Field). NCHSPC, London

Osterweiss M, Solomon F, Green M (eds) 1984 Bereavement: reactions, consequences and care. National Academy Press, Washington DC

Parkes C M 1972 Bereavement. International Universities Press, New York (now out of print)

Parkes C M 1979 Terminal care – evaluation of in-patient services at St Christopher's Hospice. Part 2: self-assessment of the service on surviving spouses. Postgraduate Medical Journal 55: 523–527

Parkes C M 1998 Traditional models and theories of grief. Bereavement Care 17(2): 21–23

Parkes C M, Weiss R S 1983 Recovery from bereavement. Basic Books, New York

Penson J, Fisher R 1995 Palliative care for people with cancer, 2nd edn. Arnold, London

Raphael B 1984 The anatomy of bereavement: a handbook for the caring professions. Hutchinson, London

Saunders C 1978 The management of terminal malignant disease. Edward Arnold, London

Smith C R 1982 Social work with the dying and the bereaved. Macmillan, London

Stroebe M S 1998 New directions in bereavement research. Palliative Medicine 12(1): 5–12

Stroebe W, Stroebe M 1987 Bereavement and health. Cambridge University Press, Cambridge

Vachon M L S, Sheldon A R, Lancee W J, Lyall W A L, Rogers J, Freeman S J J 1982 Correlates of enduring distress in bereavement; social network, life situation and personality. Psychological Medicine 12: 783–788

Walter T 1996 A new model of grief. Bereavement and Biography Mortality 1: 7–25

Walter T 1997 In: Charmaz K, Howarth G, Kellehear A (eds) The unknown country: death in Australia, Britain and the USA. Macmillan, Houndmills

Walter T 1999 On bereavement. The culture of grief. Open University Press, Buckingham

Webber J 1997 The evolving role of the Macmillan nurse. Macmillan Cancer Relief, London

Weismann A D 1979 Coping with cancer. McGraw-Hill Book Company, New York

Wendell-Moller D 1996 Confronting death: values, institutions and human mortality. Oxford University Press, Oxford

Worden W 1991 Grief counselling and grief therapy. Tavistock Routledge, London

Young M, Cullen L 1996 A good death. Routledge, London

Young M, Benjamin B, Wallis C 1963 The mortality of widowers. The Lancet 2: 454–456

FURTHER READING

Clark D 1993 (ed.) The future for palliative care. Open University Press, Buckingham

Fanslow C A 1981 Death: a natural facet of the life continuum. In Kreiger D (ed.) Foundations for holistic health nursing practices. J B Lippincott, Philadelphia, pp. 249–272

Glaser B, Strauss A 1965 Awareness of dying. Aldine, Chicago

Henley A 1986 Good practice in hospital care for the dying. King's Fund Publishing Office, London

Huber R, Gibson J W 1990 New evidence for anticipatory grief. The Hospice Journal 6: 49–67

Lugton J, Kindlen M 1999 Palliative care – the nursing role. Churchill Livingstone, Edinburgh

Samarel N 1991 Caring for life and death. Hemisphere, Washington DC

Samarel N 1995 Chapter 4. In Wass H, Neimeyer R A (eds) Dying: facing the facts, 3rd edn. Taylor and Francis, Washington DC

USEFUL INFORMATION ON BEREAVEMENT SERVICES

For parents, their families, friends and professional carers.

The Child Bereavement Trust
Director: Jenni Thomas, Brindley House,
4 Burkes Road, Beaconsfield HP9 1PB.
Tel: 01494 678088   Fax: 01494 678765

Child Death Helpline
Bereavement Services Department,
Great Ormond Street Hospital NHS Trust,
Great Ormond Street, London WC1N 3JH.
Tel: 020 7813 8551   Fax: 020 7813 8516

The Compassionate Friends
53 North Street, Bristol BS3 1EN.
Tel: 0117 966 5202   Fax: 0117 914 4368

Cruse Bereavement Care
Cruse House, 126 Sheen Road, Richmond, Surrey TW9 1UR.
Tel: 020 8940 4818   Fax: 020 8940 7638

Jewish Bereavement Counselling Service
PO Box 6748, London N3 3BX.
Tel: 020 8349 0839   Fax: 020 8349 0839

Lesbian & Gay Bereavement Project
AIDS Education Unit, Vaughan M Williams Centre, Colindale Hospital,
London NW9 5GH.
Tel: 020 8200 0511   Fax: 020 8905 9250

NAFSIYAT
Intercultural Therapy Centre, 278 Seven Sisters Road, Finsbury Park, London N4 2HY.
Tel: 020 7263 4130   Fax: 020 7561 1870

National Association of Bereavement Services
20 Norton Folgate, London E1 6DB.
Tel: 020 7247 0617   Fax: 020 7247 0617

Winston's Wish
Gloucester Royal Hospital, Great Western Road, Gloucester GL1 3NN.
Tel: 01452 394377   Fax: 01452 395656

(The authors gratefully acknowledge the Editors of the Hospice Information Service Directory 2000 who freely allowed the use of their Bereavement Section, pp. 85–87.)

11

Communication in advanced illness: challenges and opportunities

Shaun Kinghorn

INTRODUCTION

Effective communication is central to promoting high-quality palliative care. Inadequate communication may be the source of much distress for patients and their families and mitigate against adjustment to cancer and other life-threatening illnesses (Kruijver et al 2000). Effective and sensitive communication is the heart of comforting, assessment of need, expression of psychological/social spiritual distress, as well as planning for what may be perceived to be an undesirable and premature end to life. The compelling search for ways of improving communication is ongoing and there is evidence to suggest that little has improved despite a plethora of initiatives to improve the situation (Wilkinson 1991, Maguire 1999). The emergence of user-based studies also suggests there is scope for improvement in practice in meeting the informational and communication needs of patients and their families (National Cancer Alliance 1996).

Jenkins et al (1999) mention the difficulties that some medical staff have in explaining procedures such as randomised control trials to patients. The problems in discussing sensitive issues also extends to nursing staff (Wilkinson 1991, Heaven & Maguire 1996). Cancer and other life-threatening illnesses may precipitate social isolation at a time when proximal and supportive communication is seen as desirable (Bottomley 1997, Oliver 1999). Buckman (1992) reminds us that sometimes supportive communication is all that is left to give and is often administered in sub-therapeutic doses.

This chapter seeks to explore the nature of effective communication as it relates to palliative nursing, and discusses the principles that underpin the handling of awkward questions, breaking bad news and handling collusion. The focus on principles that might guide practice is supplemented by consideration of a small number of communication/counselling frameworks which may be directly relevant to the work of nurses within a palliative care context. The chapter also considers factors that influence the development of nurses' communication skills, including training, attitudes of staff, clinical supervision and evaluation of communication practice. It is acknowledged that it is not possible to cover all communication challenges and it is recommended that reference is made to associated chapters on psychological issues, loss and grief, staff support, hope and spirituality to develop a broader understanding of communication issues in advanced illness.

COMMUNICATION IN ADVANCED ILLNESS: THE CONTEXT

Recent research has intimated that little improvement is visible in the communication of nurses with cancer patients and that patients' concerns are not always elicited (Wilkinson 1991, Heaven & Maguire 1996). Such conclusions may be linked to the rapidly expanding expectations that patients and their families have and our ability to keep pace with these expectations. The expression of these expectations is receiving political and social affirmation in order that the patient can feel in control, and justified in articulating their needs. Field & Copp (1999) mention that over the last 40 years there has been a progression from a closed awareness to a more open awareness with regard to communicating with the dying. Such an assertion cannot be applied universally. Not all patients are able to clearly articulate their needs. Illness, gender, social class, fatigue and other distressing symptoms impact on the individual's capacity to express need and the emotional pain which may accompany advanced illness. It is argued that palliative care needs to be attuned to the needs of the disadvantaged dying who cannot always express their needs and fears, because of coexisting learning disabilities or mental health issues.

Advanced illness is a quagmire of painful emotions, difficult decisions and loss. Patients and their families requiring palliative care may have made contact with these services within a timeframe of weeks, or months, following an initial diagnosis. Alternatively, some require palliative care after enduring a constellation of emotionally and physically taxing therapies over a period of years. In such situations, uncertainty becomes a constant companion. The pathway, timeframes and reasons that accompany the palliative care journey are both complex and unique. An acknowledgement by the nurse that the individual has specific and unique communication needs is essential to high-quality palliative care. Lugton (1999) suggests that the individual confronted by a life-threatening illness is faced by a number of threats, which include the threat to identity and future plans; threat to social roles; threat to physical and psychosocial independence; threat to body image; threat to relationships; threat of stigma and isolation; and, finally, the threat to faith and hope. A lot of these challenges are highly dependent on the use of communication skills for assessment and resolution of concerns.

Enhancing our capacity to support patients with advanced illnesses is dependent on the development of appropriate skills and the possession of specific attitudes. This simplistic proposition fails to acknowledge the complex social context in which communicating with those with a life-threatening illness occurs. Helping patients make sense of the past and come to terms with the present and future has to acknowledge there are factors that might influence our capacity to constructively support patients and their families (Box 11.1).

COMMUNICATION CHALLENGES
Breaking bad news

Developments in the role of the nurse have led to nurses having an active role in some of the

---

Box 11.1   Factors that might create communication difficulties

- *Age of the patients* – The elderly may have hearing, sight or speech difficulties, which impacts on the expression and reception of communication needs. The age of the practitioner may also influence their attitude on how much the patient should be told regarding their illness (Gillhooly et al 1988). Communicating with the young who are dying is often considered to be a source of professional distress.

- *Factors linked to the disease or associated treatments* – These may inhibit constructive dialogue: e.g. radiotherapy or surgery to the head or neck; confusional states resulting from pharmacological interventions or the disease process.

- *The patient and family members' previous life experiences of a life-threatening illness* – These experiences may come in the form of memories of a relative or friend having had . . . or died from. . . . These experiences may form a route map for the patient to the point where they resist health care professionals' efforts to portray things as they really are.

- *Presence of distressing symptoms* – The unremitting experiences associated with breathlessness, pain, vomiting and other symptoms not only lead to emotional distress but themselves create communicating difficulties. Good symptom management is therefore a key to sustaining meaningful communication channels.

- *Blocking behaviours* – These behaviours can be initiated by nurses, patients and family members as a coping mechanism. The desire to maintain control over the present and the future may manifest itself in the patient and family blocking attempts from professionals initiating additional support. Blocking may be a reasonable coping strategy when the patient is being supported by a high number of professionals who all have a vested interest in obtaining the patient's story.

- *Cultural issues* – The various cultures which now reside in the United Kingdom have different philosophical orientations towards life and death which are likely to impact on the style and methods of communication adopted by the practitioner.

---

more challenging aspects of supporting the patient through a life-threatening illness. Although the responsibility of sharing bad news at diagnosis at present is generally in the hands of our medical colleagues, nurses are increasingly being involved in sharing bad news. Franks (1997) asserts that despite decades of attention, criticisms and coverage in the literature, bad news continues to be broken badly. The development of nurse-led clinics and a more active role in diagnostic and treatment stages of incurable illnesses will inevitably lead to nurses needing to enhance their skills in breaking bad news.

Kaye (1996) defines bad news as any information that drastically alters a patient's view of their future for the worse. In a similar vein, Buckman (1992) illustrates the destabilising nature of bad news by proposing that bad news is any news that drastically and negatively alters the patient's view of her or his future. Penson (2000) mentions that the sharing of the whole truth is often associated with taking away hope. If we get it right, the patient will never forget us; if we get it wrong, they will never forgive us (Buckman 1996). The degree of trauma associated with the news is determined by the gap between the patient's expectations and the presented truths associated with the progress of the disease. The handling of the emotions associated with 'giving bad news' can equally be distressing for the deliverer (Franks 1997). Bad news is not just linked to sharing the initial life-threatening diagnosis, it may accompany any of the following scenarios: the patient is invited to consider being admitted to a hospice; the patient is starting an opioid for pain control; the patient is informed that the side effects of drugs will promote certain disturbances in physical appearance as well as ease symptoms.

It is the patient who determines what news is bad news. The professionals involved in delivering palliative care may have their own concept of what constitutes bad news; these perceptions may not be totally congruent with the patient. This is aptly demonstrated in the following situation, which illustrates that bad news may not be as emotionally toxic as living with uncertainty. Upon arriving on duty, the

- The individual may not have the skills to handle the question and the subsequent issues.
- The question may be accompanied by intense emotion, such as anxiety, anger and other forms of distress.
- For the nurse the question may rekindle powerful personal memories of past difficult situations, both personal and professional.

There are of course no stock phrases or answers which can adequately respond to such questions. The answer lies in the sensitive application of the following principles which are designed to elicit the most pressing concerns beneath the question. Firstly, it is important to:

(a) Acknowledge that the question is important to the individual and merits your undivided attention.
(b) Use skilful questioning, preferably with open questions, to help facilitate the ventilation of feelings and elicit what the real issues are.
(c) Listen intently throughout.
(d) Summarise what has been said to clarify the nature of the problem.
(e) Decide the appropriate response.

Once again, exploration precedes response. The application of these principles is manifest in the situation given in Case study 11.2.

Perhaps the application of the following principles to Case study 11.2 may help. It is not suggested this should be a template for every similar situation, but nevertheless it is there to illustrate how awkward questions require systematic exploration to ensure the response is helpful to the patient.

(a) Acknowledge that the question is important to the individual and merits your time

You could allow a little silence to pass by if nothing further comes; then make sure John is in a quiet, comfortable position where there is some privacy. It may be appropriate to repeat the question back to John and ask him to offer some background to the question.

(b) Use skilful questioning, preferably with open questions, to help facilitate the ventilation of feelings and elicit what the real issues are

Questions which may help promote further discussion could include:

- What's your impression of what the future holds?
- What would you want to do with the time you now have?
- How can we help?
- You look . . . ?

(c) Listen intently throughout

There is a possibility that John may expand on his awareness of lost future opportunities and the total pain of being confronted with a time-limiting illness. During this period the carers develop greater insight into the real issues and perhaps witness John coming to terms with the realities of the future. This may include not seeing the arrival of his first grandchild. Aspirations when verbalised by the patients can then be confirmed or highlighted as being difficult.

(d) Summarise what has been said to clarify the nature of the problem

In the outpouring of concerns and emotion which may accompany the handling of awkward

---

CASE STUDY 11.2

HANDLING AWKWARD QUESTIONS

John is a 55-year-old man, who has a carcinoma of the colon, being cared for in your surgical unit. He has secondary deposits in his liver and has recently undergone palliative chemotherapy. He is married with two daughters aged 24 and 21 who no longer live at home with their mother Grace. Melinda, John and Grace's older daughter, is expecting a baby in 3 months' time. John is fatigued, anxious and complaining of back pain and upper abdominal pain. You are helping him get ready one morning when he starts to mutter: 'I am not getting any better'. This quiet statement is followed by: 'How long have I got?'. How are you going to respond?

questions a mini-summary helps ensure what is being presented by the patient has been correctly interpreted. In this instance, the following example may be appropriate.

John, we started by you asking me a fairly direct question in which you asked 'how long have I got?' You have mentioned that there is much you wish to do and have expressed concerns over the fact that you may never see your first grandchild. It appears that this may be your biggest concern as well as concerns over how Grace, your wife, will cope.

(e) Decide the appropriate response

In this situation, in view of John's continual deterioration, it is probable that he may not see the arrival of his grandchild. This uncertainty cannot be replaced with false reassurances. What can be offered is the assistance from the social worker and the rest of the team, that John, at his pace, may develop a memory box in order that he can be remembered by his first grandchild. Further assistance and support can be offered to help him and his wife to plan for the future, whatever shape or form that might take.

Situations like the above place high demands on the communication skills of the practitioner and it is advisable that support mechanisms such as clinical supervision are essential where such situations are frequently encountered.

COMMUNICATING AT THE END OF LIFE: WHICH FRAMEWORKS?

The development of specialist posts in palliative nursing in a variety of settings has led to the requirement of an advanced set of communication competencies. Consistency in delivering advanced practice may require the nurse to base the helping relationship on counselling/communication frameworks. A significant portion of the chapter has considered practice which is guided by principles. These principles have to a greater extent emerged in order to guide the practitioner and cope with the emotional chaos which

> **Reflection point**
>
> List the awkward questions/queries from patients and their families you have found difficult to handle and consider what makes these questions difficult to handle.

may accompany breaking bad news, handling awkward questions and preparing the patient and family for death. Using these principles is appropriate in handling short-duration communication issues. In some instances it is necessary to base practice on counselling frameworks which may help patients resolve past, current and anticipated problems related to the threat of a limited life span. Counselling frameworks can not only provide frameworks for practice but can also offer preferred attributes that may facilitate a genuine helping relationship which can be the basis of helping patients adjust to the challenges associated with a limited life span.

John Heron (1993) promotes the notion of the helper as someone who can support, enable and promote well-being in the individual. It is further suggested that the helper may have five key attributes:

- warm concern and acceptance for another
- openness and atunement to the other's experiential reality
- a grasp of what the other needs for his/her essential flourishing
- an ability to facilitate the flourishing of such needs in the right manner at the right time
- an authentic presence.

Heron's assertion that the helper has to possess desirable attributes is supported by Bailey & Wilkinson (1998) who conducted a study involving 36 patients with advanced cancer designed to elicit patients' views on nurses' communication skills. Twenty-seven patients suggested that good verbal and non-verbal skills, demonstration of approachable personal attributes and having knowledge of their subject were highly desirable. The attributes mentioned in essence form the core values which underpin some of the six categories of counselling intervention. The creative communicator is one who can successfully reconcile desirable personal attributes with established counselling/communication frameworks. The application of Heron's theory of human nature can be more adequately explored in a paper by Liossi & Mystakidou (1997). Heron describes the six categories as having the following dimensions:

Authoritative

1. *Prescriptive* – A prescriptive intervention seeks to direct the behaviour of the client, usually behaviour that is outside the practitioner–client relationship.
2. *Informative* – An informative intervention seeks to impart knowledge and information to the client.
3. *Confronting* – A confronting intervention seeks to raise the client's consciousness about some limiting attitude or behaviour of which they are relatively unaware.

Facilitative

4. *Cathartic* – A cathartic intervention seeks to enable the client to discharge, to abreact a painful emotion, primarily grief, fear and anger.
5. *Catalytic* – A catalytic intervention seeks to elicit self-discovery, self-directed living, learning and problem-solving in the client.
6. *Supportive* – A supportive intervention seeks to affirm the worth and value of the client's person, qualities, attitudes or actions.

The authoritative interventions are very much lodged in a hierarchical domain, whereas the facilitative interventions are more dependent on the client leading the agenda, discharging feelings and discerning the nature of the problem and potential solutions. Case study 11.3 illustrates the scope of using this module in a palliative care situation. It is acknowledged that the timing and appropriate sequencing of these interventions needs to be mediated by Brian and his family.

Applying the six-category intervention model to Case study 11.3, it is clear that the facilitative interventions will need to be consistently applied by all staff to create a climate of trust and reassuring presence. Unconditional positive regard and calm communication will help nurture a rapport with family members.

Supportive. Staff should affirm the worth of Jenny and her family, and elicit the depth of suffering she and her family are experiencing. Since Brian is visiting his wife regularly this will affect his capacity to maintain a regular income. This will be a source of concern for Jenny. Her fear of dying during a panic attack and the role shift accompanying dependence 'on her family' for care may be concerns which could be expressed.

Cathartic. Both Jenny and her family may have concealed a wide range of fears relating to the present and the future. It is likely that each member will have their own emotional profile which may include anger, uncertainty and anxiety: no-one may want to unburden to another member of the family. As a result, the hurt and distress may be carefully contained. The therapeutic value of simply listening to patients ventilating their feelings which may be manifest in tears, shouting or anger cannot be underestimated. Heron acknowledges the centrality of unconditional positive regard as a key to the door in sometimes unleashing painful

---

CASE STUDY 11.3

INTERVENTION MODEL

Jenny is a 51-year-old lady who has advanced carcinoma of the lung. She has been recently admitted to the hospice for pain and symptom control. Jenny has been married to her husband Brian for 26 years. Brian is self-employed, running his own electrical contracting business. Jenny and Brian have two sons, Grant aged 17 and David aged 25. David lives 4 hours' drive away and is married to Sheila. They are expecting their second child in 3 months' time. While at home Jenny was becoming increasingly dependent on her family to meet her daily needs. Prior to admission, Brian and her younger son, Grant, were looking after Jenny with assistance from the district nurse and the GP. Jenny is anxious and nocturnal panic attacks have been an emerging problem.

emotions. It is often the case that during these out-bursts the real fears emerge. Statements such as: 'You look close to tears' . . . 'You look angry' . . . 'How are you coping with what is happening to you?' . . . may offer an opportunity for the practitioner to unlock the door. Jenny may be upset at the possibility that she may not be remembered as a grandmother. In a similar vein, David and Sheila may have reflected on the possibility that their children may never see their grandmother.

Informative. The emergence of panic attacks may have been precipitated by fear of dying in her sleep. It may be helpful for the practitioner to take time to explain the antecedents to panic attacks and that they can be controlled. There is also the possibility that Jenny may want to know how exactly she will die and seek the advice of a practitioner on how appropriate it would be to have family members present 'when that time' arrives. Information regarding the availability of services which could support Jenny and her family at home in the future could be offered.

Catalytic. A catalytic intervention aims to seek solutions in what may appear to be seemingly impossible situations. Utilising this approach, the team could help Jenny and her husband look towards the future and 'get things in order' such as finances, funeral, etc. With this intervention the pace at which issues are explored requires delicate treatment in order that Jenny is empowered with a sense of control. Catalytic interventions can be helpful in ensuring that Jenny might be able to explore ways in which she would want to be remembered in the future.

Confronting. Palliative care is often perceived to be a 'gentle' discipline which does not embrace confrontation as a core value. Nevertheless, it may be appropriate in a sensitive manner for the practitioner to reflect back to Jenny or her family the consequences of actions which may not be conducive to a peaceful death.

Not all the six interventions may be indicated in every given situation, neither is it the responsibility of one practitioner to utilise all the strategies. The social worker may find that they are 'on the receiving end' of Brian's and other family members' distress, whereas the nurse and med-ical team may be principally involved in informative/supportive interventions.

NON-DIRECTIVE FRAMEWORKS: THE ONLY OPTION?

Other frameworks, including the use of cognitive behavioural therapy – which has received increasing attention concerning its application to palliative care – could also handle the case of Jenny. Although research into its application in a cancer/palliative care situation is in its infancy the evidence for its use in handling depression and anxiety is compelling (Blackburn & Davidson 1990, Enright 1997, Moorey et al 1998). Anxiety and depression are common adjustment reactions to living under the cloud of a life-threatening illness.

With cancer now affecting approximately one in three people, it is inevitable that carers may experience cognitions which are based on the experience of a relative dying with cancer. It is commonplace to a see a distressed relative who at some stage observed the death of a close family member.

The use of this framework may shed light on the reasons underpinning nurses' difficulty in eliciting key concerns of patients and family members. Heaven & Maguire (1996) argue that nurses lack the therapeutic skills to assess patients' individual concerns and problems. They concluded that simple skills training is unlikely to change behaviour. The drive towards encouraging nurses to be active listeners and use non-directive approaches may have contributed to this situation.

What are the key features of cognitive behavioural therapy (CBT)? This therapy is a problem oriented approach, which aims to help the patient identify and modify dysfunctional thought, assumption and patterns of behaviour (Enright 1997). Foster & McLellan (2000) illustrate the relevance of this model to palliative care by mentioning that cognitive behavioural interventions are brief in nature and solution-focused. It is a therapeutic approach that encourages the practitioner to focus on the key concerns of the clients and how the thoughts associated with these concerns impact on their emotions.

Box 11.4   Cognitive behavioural therapy

1. *Time limited* – programmes usually last a maximum of 4 months. Each session being 1 hour in duration.
2. *Agenda/structure* – each session is guided by an agenda to utilise time to its maximum use. Each session usually lasts 1 hour.
3. *Problem-oriented* – the therapist and patient focus on defining and solving the presenting problems.
4. *Ahistorical* – deals with the here and now without recourse to the distant past history of the patient.
5. *Scientific methods* – the approach in establishing the boundaries of a problem and potential solution utilises collecting data; formulating hypotheses; and evaluating results.
6. *Homework* – the patient is often given homework to verify assumptions regarding negative thoughts and the evidence to support their existence. Proactive use of cognitive skills is often a feature of homework.
7. *Collaboration* – patient and therapist work together to solve problems.
8. *Active and directive* – the therapist is often called up to be directive and didactic, sometimes in the quest to define the problem and resolve identified problems.
9. *Use of Socratic questioning* – the principal mode of questioning which aims to help the patient identify underlying thoughts and develop alternative solutions or modify opinions.
10. *Openness* – this process of cognitive therapy is explicit and open.

Blackburn & Davidson (1990) illustrate the key features of this approach (Box 11.4).

Those concerned over the challenging nature of this intervention will be reassured that the client-centred attributes of empathy, warmth, genuineness and understanding are seen as desirable with this approach. Blackburn & Davidson (1990) mention that these attributes alone are insufficient to bring about resolution of anxiety and depression.

Although it is not possible to provide an extensive review of the application of this approach, it is possible to speculate that the principles of cognitive therapy sensitively applied may be of value in handling the following issues/questions:

- Panic attacks, when the patient expresses he feels he is going to die during an episode of breathlessness.

- Handling collusion: 'it will be best if we don't tell her as she just won't cope'.
- 'There's nothing to live for now.'
- 'Don't bring my granddaughter to see me, she will very soon forget I ever existed.'
- 'I suppose I will just die in agony as my father did.'

Individuals experience psychological distress when they face a threat to their key interests (McLeod 1993). The threat of cancer and its associated treatments can be classed as a threat that can ultimately lead to the individual having difficulty in turning off distorted thinking. Not all the above situations will merit a full therapeutic programme and the issue of limited life span may make this improbable to enter such a contract. The application of the principles of cognitive therapy may bring a more satisfactory resolution rather than purely entering a non-directive dialogue.

In view of the limited life expectancy of many patients receiving palliative care and the drift towards developing palliative care outpatients' services it is suggested that further exploration on the role of CBT as a therapeutic approach merits further consideration.

The practice of encouraging practitioners to enrol on 'counselling courses' as a prerequisite for undertaking a specialist role has been a feature of specialist practitioner preparation over the last decade. This drive was advocated without the benefit of research to validate the appropriateness of such preparation on patients requiring palliative care.

The notion that the nurse or any other practitioner needing a framework to guide effective practice is well illustrated in research supporting the use of cognitive behavioural therapy. Moorey et al (1998) in a study involving cancer patients compared two psychological treatments: namely, adjuvant psychological therapy (APT) and supportive counselling. It was concluded that APT produced greater changes in anxiety and adjustment to cancer. APT is very much based on the principles of CBT. Although research into its application in a cancer/palliative care situation is in its infancy the evidence for its use in handling depression and anxiety within mental health is well established. As noted earlier, Foster & McLellan (2000) mention that cognitive behavioural interventions are brief and solution-focused. CBT is a therapeutic approach which encourages the practitioner to focus on the key concerns of the patient and how the thoughts associated with these concerns impact on their emotions. Once the 'thoughts' that trigger emotional responses to the threat of cancer and/or its treatment are identified, this therapeutic approach can have a clearer focus and therefore tackle issues, which can be eased within a limited timespan. Application of CBT is well established in the management of anxiety and depression within the sphere of mental health services. In view of the limited life expectancy of clients receiving palliative care, the spotlight is increasingly being focused on approaches such as CBT.

DEVELOPING COMMUNICATION PRACTICE: THE OPTIONS

The issue of enhancing communication practice via training with seriously ill patients has received considerable attention (Wilkinson 1991, Heaven & Maguire 1996, Wilkinson et al 1998, Booth et al 1999). Teaching which raises awareness of issues surrounding death and dying may facilitate an increased willingness to approach the dying but not positively impact on eliciting patient/family concerns or improve competence in handling awkward questions.

Heaven & Maguire (1996) mention that simple skills training is insufficient to alter clinical behaviour. This conclusion emerged from a study involving 44 hospice nurses who participated in an evaluation of a 10-week communication course, which had a particular focus on the nurse's ability to elicit patients' concerns. The programme was very much based on the skills of assessment. These skills were evaluated by analysis of audiotaped conversations with patients. It was concluded that there was a lack of improvement in the outcome of communication, which was demonstrated by the fact that before and after training nurses identified

less than 40% of the concerns that patients raised. Since hospice care encompasses a multi-professional ethos, it is possible that the socialisation of hospice nurses mitigates against them taking sole responsibility for eliciting total concerns. It is possible, despite the impact of trying, that they may be cognitively attuned to specific concerns and conscious that it is the combined efforts of the whole team which produces a comprehensive picture of the patient/family concerns.

Wilkinson et al (1998) evaluated the value of nurse–patient communication in a palliative care programme, which involved 110 nurses completing a 26-hour training programme over a 6-month period. The training programme had a broader base than the study previously cited, and included knowledge and attitudes as well as assessment skills. The content of the programme included coverage of topics such as counselling skills, loss, grief and bereavement; body image; and anxiety and depression. A pre-course and post-course audiotape was used to elicit competence in patient assessment skills. Also students had the option of formal assessment by conducting a written critique of their skills. It was concluded that there was a statistically significant improvement in assessment skills from pre-test to post-test scores, with 90% of participants having increased their scores. Audiotape recordings, self-critique and feedback sessions were described as being the most valuable elements of the programme.

It would appear if there is to be a significant development in nurses' skills, training programmes will need to include feedback, review of audiotape/videotape situations and the opportunity for the practitioner to examine his/her own skills and attitudes in relation to patients requiring palliative care. These difficulties are clearly compounded by uncertainty regarding the type of competencies that need to be established in guiding the novice and the expert practitioner alike. Husband et al (2000) highlight the need for cancer training and education using a competency-based approach. One of the nine competencies specified in the paper was that of communication. Using the competency-based approach, the novice practitioner could evolve from merely being able to identify a patient and family in distress to a higher level skill of delivering a range of systematic therapeutic interventions which may have a demonstrable effect on reducing anxiety and depression. The identification of competencies and the designation of programmes to meet these competencies may contribute to resolving the problems highlighted by previous research in nurses failing to elicit patients' and family members' primary concerns.

Although research indicates the positive influence some training packages can have, sustainable change and communication skills are likely to be enhanced by a programme of clinical supervision. Clinical supervision has an established history in social work, counselling and mental health nursing. In view of the likelihood that the nurse in palliative care is confronted by difficult communication scenarios, the practice of clinical supervision would seem commensurate with the development of high-quality clinical practice. The emotional labour of palliative nursing is graphically represented in a study by Jones (1999), who cites the case of a Macmillan nurse who mentions that: 'the patient will look at me without a single word and convey the message I know that you know'. Jones (1999) further mentions that supervision can help the nurse make sense of complex feelings, which may accompany difficult communication issues, and provides an opportunity to process and refine feelings, thoughts and actions which emerge from professional practice. In essence, palliative care nurses may be participating in momentous experiences in the lives of patients and their families (Jones 1997). Involvement in such experiences is not without its problems. Concerning the hazards of helping, Hawkins & Shohet (1997) mention that we may find ourselves in a position where we consider ourselves to be helpers rather than a channel for help. Such self-awareness is essential if the professional is to be consistent in maintaining his/her effectiveness as a communicator with the seriously ill. Such awareness can be facilitated in a variety of ways, including clinical supervision.

A significant portion of the palliative care nurse's role is conducted in one-to-one situations: the process of the developing nurse–patient relationship may take place beyond the gaze of other colleagues. Alternatively, physical care for the highly dependent may be given in twos, whereas handling sensitive communication may be handled alone. This lone practice is commensurate with privacy and the promotion of a climate where the patient may freely express fears and major concerns. It is this scenario which creates a situation where the nurse may feel: 'How do I know if I got it right?', 'Did I say the right thing' or 'Perhaps I could have listened more'. It is argued that clinical supervision is essential if communication practice is to be enhanced.

Developments in communicating with the seriously ill could be facilitated by palliative care staff having a more active role in auditing practice. The King's Fund (Walker et al 1996) published guidelines for delivering a cancer diagnosis. The guidelines primarily focus on the primary/secondary interface, the communication of bad news and organisational issues. Such a document is welcome in view of the ever-mounting concerns that patients and families express regarding lack of communication. Even though we might provide training programmes and have started to instigate clinical supervision, the development of a communication audit will help palliative care nurses ascertain the quality of communication they offer to patients and their families.

CONCLUSION

As we move into a new millennium, nurses will be increasingly entrusted with the responsibility of playing an active role in handling some of the more difficult communication issues which have up until now been the domain of medical staff. The development of nurse-led clinics will place new demands on the communication skills of nurses. Such responsibilities need to be accompanied by adequate

> **Reflection point**
>
> In what ways could you and the team you work with more effectively communicate with patients and their families?

preparation, which is based on clearly defined competencies, evaluation and ongoing supervision. These prerequisites are essential in facilitating excellence in communicating with the seriously ill. The current drive to network with other specialties and disciplines is encouraging palliative care nursing to consider other models of supportive communication, such as cognitive behavioural therapy. Being equipped with the skills to evaluate the application of such frameworks within a palliative care context will help enhance the evidence base of palliative nursing.

REFERENCES

Bailey K, Wilkinson S 1998 Patients' views on nurses' communication skills: a pilot study. International Journal of Palliative Nursing 4(6): 300–305

Booth K, Maguire P, Hillier V F 1999 Measurement of communication skills in cancer care: myth or reality? Journal of Advanced Nursing 30(5): 1073–1079

Blackburn I, Davidson K 1990 Cognitive therapy for depression and anxiety. Blackwell Scientific, Oxford

Bottomley A 1997 Social support and the cancer patient: a need for clarity. European Journal of Cancer Care 6: 72–77

Buckman R 1992 How to break bad news: a guide for health care professionals. Papermac, Basingstoke

Buckman R 1996 Talking to patients about cancer: no excuse for not doing it now. British Medical Journal 313: 699–700

Enright S 1997 Cognitive behavioral therapy. British Medical Journal 314: 1811–1822

Fallowfield L, Ford S, Lewis S 1995 No news is not good news: information preferences of patients with cancer. Psycho-Oncology 4: 197–202

Faulkener A 1998 When the news is bad: a guide for health professionals. Stanley Thornes Ltd, Cheltenham

Field D, Copp G 1999 Communication and awareness about dying in the 1990s. Palliative Medicine 13: 459–468

Foster L W, McLellan L 2000 Cognition and cancer experience: clinical applications. Cancer Pract 8(1): 25–31

Franks A 1997 Breaking bad news and the challenge of communication. European Journal of Palliative Care 4(2): 61–66

Gillhooly M, Berkeley J, McCann K, Gibling F, Murray K 1988 Truth telling with dying cancer patients. Palliative Medicine 2: 64–71

Hawkins P, Shohet R 1997 Supervision in the helping professions. Open University Press, Milton Keynes

Heron J 1993 Helping the client: a creative practical approach. Sage Publications, London

Heaven K, Maguire P 1996 Training hospice nurses to elicit patient concerns. Journal of Advanced Nursing 23: 280–286

Husband G, Banks-Howe J, Boal L, Hodgson D 2000 A competency-based tool for education. European Journal of Cancer Care 9: 36–40

Jenkins V A, Fallowfield L J, Souhami A, Sawtell M 1999 How do doctors explain RCTs to their patients. European Journal of Cancer 35(8): 1187–1193

Jones A 1997 A 'bonding between strangers': a palliative model of clinical supervision. Journal of Advanced Nursing 26: 1028–1035

Jones A 1999 'A heavy and blessed experience': a psychoanalytic study of community Macmillan nurses and their roles in serious illness and palliative care. Journal of Advanced Nursing 30(6): 1297–1303

Kaye P 1996 Breaking bad news: a ten step approach. EPL Publications, Northampton

Kendrick K 1994 Ethical pathways in cancer and palliative care. In: David J Cancer care prevention, treatment and palliation. Chapman and Hall, London

Kruijver I, Kerkstra A, Bensing J, Van der Wiel H 2000 Nurse/patient communication in cancer care. A review of the literature. Cancer Nursing 23(1): 20–31

Liossi C, Mystakidou K 1997 Heron's theory of human needs in palliative care. European Journal of Palliative Care 4(1): 32–35

Litcher I 1978 Communication in cancer care. Churchill Livingstone, Edinburgh

Lugton J 1999 Support processes in palliative care. In: Lugton J, Kindlen M (eds) Palliative care: the nurses role. Churchill Livingstone, Edinburgh

McLeod J 1993 An introduction to counselling. Open University Press, Buckingham

Maguire P 1999 Improving communication with cancer patients. European Journal of Cancer 35(10): 1415–1422

Moorey S, Greer S, Bliss J, Law M 1998 A comparison of adjuvant psychological therapy and supportive counselling in patients with cancer. Psycho-Oncology 7: 218–228

Morley C 1997 The use of denial by patients with cancer. Professional Nurse 12(5): 380–381

National Cancer Alliance 1996 'Patient-centered cancer services'?: what patients say. NCA Publications, Oxford

Oliver G 1999 The Robert Tiffany Annual Lecture 14th June 1999: Moving Oncology Nursing Forward, an Agenda for the 21st Century. European Journal of Cancer Care 8: 192–197

Penson J 2000 A hope is not a promise: fostering hope within palliative care. International Journal of Palliative Nursing 6(2): 94–97

their illness and its progression, waiting for someone to react in the context of the real facts in order to help them comes to terms with things. Each person shares some responsibility for either maintaining or breaking the unwritten code of avoidance, and the transition to an open awareness may be sudden or gradual.

As 24-hour carers, nurses are in a unique situation to be party to this change in perception and can help facilitate its smooth transition where possible. The nursing role here is dependent on the trust and rapport which has been built with the respective family members. It places the nurse potentially at the centre of this major life crisis and all the consequent cathartic emotional release that may go with it. The opportunity to shape and influence the coping strategies of the patient and family at this crucial and vulnerable time is immense and is surely at the very core of palliative nursing practice. There are no guarantees of course and it is just as possible to hinder the situation rather than help it. The key word here is opportunity.

The psychological reaction of the nurse

When nurses care for the dying they know that they are expected to provide not only physical care but also understanding, comfort and emotional support for the patient and their family. Indeed this holistic emphasis on care is clearly emphasised in a number of reports and definitions of palliative care (EAPC 1989, WHO 1990, NCHSPCS 1995). However, our culture tends to emphasise youth, life and avoidance of the taboo subject of death (Aries 1993). Nurse training itself has a high emphasis on all aspects of individual health maintenance, as one would expect, and new nurses learn very quickly about the complexities of defining and promoting health from both an academic and an individual perspective, until, that is, they are introduced in the classroom to the psychological care of someone who is dying and caring for their family. The looks of astonishment and worry are almost universal, regardless of age and life experience. Perhaps not surprisingly they had understood that one day they would encounter death as part of the nurse's role, but did not see it as such an integral part of care, and were disturbed by the very thought of dealing with it so soon and indeed so often. What is easily forgotten is that as nurses we are exposed to the same media representations of life and the same role models, and share in the same cultural values and beliefs as those people we are asked to look after. We live in the same communities and conduct our lives in similar ways; the only difference is that these people are facing the fact of their own mortality. It is a sobering thought and one which nurses from all areas are naturally reluctant to face. Why should we, after all; we all harbour expectations of a long and healthy life.

There can be a sense that being a professional carer confers some passive immunity from confronting issues to do with personal death. Educational and life experience tells us that death is something that happens to others and on the television and yet we are expected to face this fundamental issue directly in order to deliver quality nursing care. We do know, however, that it is not dealing with difficult issues that causes burnout in staff; rather, it is the lack of involvement and distancing from the patient which is the main contributor (Benner & Wrubel 1989). Avoidance of involvement with the dying actually contributes to one of the patient's major problems: i.e. loneliness and isolation. The phrase: 'How will I cope?' is just as true for the nurse as it is for the patient and family. How then can this be resolved?

The first step is for the nurse to consciously become aware of her feelings and behaviours in dealing with the dying. Few nurses have come to terms with their own finality and are at peace with the concept of death. As a result they may inadvertently project their fears onto the patient. There is a useful five-stage structure (Box 12.1) described by Harper (1977) which looks at the way nurses adjust to the psychological trauma of palliative nursing and can help a person understand more clearly what is happening to them.

This structure is not intended to be prescriptive, and many of us may find ourselves operating at varying levels of compassion and competence

CASE STUDY 12.1

A PATIENT IN HOSPITAL

Anne was first diagnosed with cancer 3 years ago and underwent a mastectomy. Following the operation, she undertook a course of adjuvant chemotherapy which she received on an outpatient basis. Despite the loss of her hair which concerned her greatly, her recovery was steady. On a routine 6-monthly visit to her consultant, she complained of lower back pain and a swollen left eye. Soon after, she was admitted for investigations, which revealed large metastases in her lower spine and one in her left orbit. Radiotherapy was given and, following a full assessment for her pain, an extensive regimen was prescribed.

Within a week her condition began to deteriorate and her daughter Rachel and husband and son Alan had travelled some 200 miles from their homes in Scotland to be by her side. Anne was well informed of her situation and presented as a stoical, smiling and uncomplaining lady, with great strength of character. Her determination to adopt a positive approach throughout her illness had clearly helped her and to some extent her children, who now had to deal with the very real prospect of their mother's death.

Alan, in particular, was finding it very distressing and was often angry about his impotence to change the situation his mother was in. He would change the subject whenever his mother wished to discuss her illness and would excuse himself from the room whenever he could. He clearly did not know what to do or to say and this made him feel uneasy when he was sitting by her bed. The key nurse involved quietly suggested that he try holding her hand and reassured him that he need not always have to say anything.

His sister Rachel used her husband for support and appeared to be coping better with the reality of her mother's impending death. It was her now emaciated body and badly swollen eye which caused them much distress. Anne realised this herself and would weep quietly after they had left. It was important therefore for the staff to be available to be with her at this sensitive time. In small ways both children became involved in their mother's care, by providing her with her favourite music to listen to, a regular supply of magazines and her own night clothes and make-up. They would often read to her, selecting brief items of news. Anne asked few questions of the staff, and was an articulate intelligent lady who had worked in a high-powered job for most of her life. Her need for accurate information was therefore clearly expressed many times.

After several days, she began to slip in and out of consciousness, with occasional moments of lucidity, and she died peacefully one lunchtime with her family at her side. Alan broke down in tears almost immediately and was comforted by his sister. They stayed at their mother's side for some 20 minutes saying their goodbyes and thanked the staff before they left. Alan commented that he felt satisfied that he had been able to communicate with his mother and appreciated being able to be there and help a little.

---

on a daily basis: such is life. What it does do, however, is to give us a guide by which to judge our professional and personal effectiveness in delivering a true palliative approach.

Box 12.1   Five-stage structure (Harper 1977)

1. Attaining knowledge of practice and loss.
2. Facing the emotional trauma of dealing with loss itself.
3. Deciding whether to 'grow' or 'go' with the job, i.e. stay with these encounters or simply leaving the job.
4. Actively reflecting and learning about oneself from the experience of dealing with death and developing our self-awareness.
5. Developing a sense of deep compassion and empathy in our care, which comes over strongly to the patient and family.

EXPLORING THE PRACTICE-BASED REALITY

A patient in hospital

This is explored in Case study 12.1.

Research-based analysis

There are a number of valuable learning points which arise from Case study 12.1 that can shape and influence our nursing practice.

• Anne's body image and perception of self is clearly a major nursing concern. Not only has she lost her breast and hair, but also her face is becoming disfigured due to the swelling in her left eye. Studies of the mental health of women who have undergone mastectomy and chemotherapy (Maguire et al 1980) have shown that body image and sexuality are inextricably linked and the psychological impact is considerable. There are two main factors here:

1. Body perception – how individuals visualise their body.
2. Body attitude – how individuals value their body and their feelings towards it (Cronan 1993).

A change of body image may also be defined as a loss of psychological self, including loss of self-concept, self-esteem and self-identity. From a cultural perspective there can be a loss of social role and identity (Burt 1995). In Anne's case this was significant.

- The psychological reaction of the son Alan and daughter Rachel to their mother's fate can be understood better by reference to research into grief and loss, such as that by Parkes (1986), who describes a four-phase approach; Kubler-Ross (1970), who used a five-stage approach; Worden (1991), who used a four-task approach; and Giaquinta (1977), who talked of five adaptation stages with families. Each of these eminent authors offers us a sound conceptual explanation for the behaviour exhibited. They base their theories around the process or linear approach to understanding such major life crises and their work has made a major contribution in this area. The shock, despair, denial, anger and sense of impotence that Alan felt coupled with his eventual reconciling to the situation as he adapted are all indicative patterns of normal behaviour, which the nurse can place into context for Alan.

- Anne's stoical reaction to her illness is very culturally contextual to British society. When Murgatroyd & Wolf (1982) examined the sociology of death they commented that it is rarely openly talked about in Western society. The focus within a family tends to be on the organisation of the practicalities and coping with day-to-day life rather than dealing with feelings, anxieties and thoughts. Clearly, all members of this family had a need to support each other in whatever way they could, and it is up to the nurse to facilitate this.

- The need for the nurse to foster better communication both verbally and non-verbally was of paramount importance to this family if they were to attempt to come to terms with the impact of Anne's impending death. Any serious illness or condition where recovery is unlikely or impossible serves to remind people of their own mortality and increases their sense of fear and vulnerability (Maguire & Faulkner 1988). There has been a vast multitude of appropriate research into the way nurses communicate with the dying and their relatives. Much of this highlights the limitations of busy clinical environments and the impediments which mitigate against its success (Field 1989).

- The use of touch, that most basic form of communication, was evident in this study. Touch has the ability to convey a huge amount of reassurance and empathy (Le May 1986). Anne was very concerned about Alan, who was younger than his sister and had been living at home until very recently. Encouraging him to hold onto his mother's hand may have also helped to reduce Anne's anxieties. We should never underestimate the potency of this form of non-verbal communication with another person (Cassey 1994, Davies 1994).

- The tears from Alan can be difficult to deal with, as there is an expectation in most Western societies that men will remain in charge of their emotions in most situations (Staudacher 1991). We also know quite clearly that encouraging and allowing the expression of such grief is a healthy thing (Worden 1991). There is therefore a need to allow Alan time and space to express himself as

---

Box 12.2   Unexpected behaviours (Staudacher 1991)

- Lose control over a situation
- Openly cry
- Be afraid or dependent
- Be insecure, anxious or passive
- Express loneliness, sadness or depression
- Express the need for love and affection
- Be playful and touch other men
- Exhibit what are considered typically 'feminine' characteristics

he sees fit, and to understand the psychological contradictions that confront men in these sensitive situations. In her book *Men and Grief* Staudacher (1991) considers that Western men are under considerable cultural pressure to behave in a certain way when dealing with grief and cites a range of the most common behaviours which are not expected (Box 12.2).

While these somewhat unrealistic expectations may make life bearable in the short term, they can make the successful resolution of loss a difficult issue. Allowing the family to stay at the bedside to say their goodbyes is a very positive and supportive part of the nurse's role. It can, nevertheless, be difficult to achieve in a busy acute clinical environment, due to the incessant pressure on bed occupancy. Gone are the days when a body would be left on a ward for up to 6 or more hours to allow relatives to visit. There is anecdotal evidence to suggest that 1 hour is more common today, and even that is in jeopardy at times.

A patient at home

This is explored in Case study 12.2.

Research-based analysis

- The district nursing team recognised that unhurried visits early in the terminal illness

---

CASE STUDY 12.2

A PATIENT AT HOME

Maureen was a 58-year-old lady who lived in a small rural village with her husband Tom and several dogs. She was diagnosed with multiple sclerosis some 3 years ago and took early retirement from her job as a result. Up until 3 months ago her mobility and control over her life had been good, but following their return from a short holiday abroad she had begun to deteriorate rapidly, and was now housebound and very weak. The district nurses visited twice a week to help her to shower and provide some psychosocial support. She was a lady who valued her independence and privacy; therefore during the visits it was important for the nurse to maximise the opportunity to talk to her about her situation, her fears and coping strategies. Inevitably, therefore, the time spent in the bathroom was sometimes over an hour. Maureen's husband was very supportive and grateful for the help. As the main carer he was frequently exhausted, and very protective towards his wife.

Often he could hear laughter coming from the bathroom, which he found disconcerting; as for example one day the zip on Maureen's dress burst and she commented: 'I've come this far without a diet and I'm not starting now for anyone'. At most visits after the shower the nurse would sit and take coffee with them both. The conversation revolved around grandchildren, parenting, social activities and, when appropriate, Maureen's illness. There was a comfortable and respectful honesty between all concerned.

As she deteriorated, her bed was brought downstairs to a lounge room that overlooked their large and well-tended garden. This gave Maureen the opportunity to be near her dogs which she adored and to be close to natural light and to her much cherished garden. They had a wide circle of friends who used to call round, but these visits began to diminish as she got progressively worse.

The visits from the nurse therefore were much more than merely attending to practical tasks; they became a 'lifeline to normality' as Tom put it and a chance also to speak honestly to someone independent about the attitudes of their friends and their sense of abandonment.

As Maureen's death became imminent the visits increased, and on one occasion she was particularly low. She spoke not about herself, but the effect her condition was having on Tom's mental health. Although they were open with each other about her condition she noticed that he was becoming very joking and yet distant at the same time, which she felt was out of character. His attitude and demeanour changed towards the nurse and he kept conversations very brief and dismissive of the situation approaching.

Maureen died a peaceful death about 10 days later, with her husband and dogs by her side. The district nurse visited soon after and encountered a tirade of verbal hostility from Tom which was mixed with many regrets. The nurse tried to calm the situation down, but without success and left soon after. She visited again 2 days later and found a tearful, remorseful and rather drunk Tom, who apologised for his previous behaviour. The nurse made some strong coffee, sat down with Tom and listened carefully over the next hour to his story. At times he sank into tearful despair, alternating with an appropriate light-hearted comment about Maureen's life and her habits. As she left that day Tom squeezed her hand gently, smiled and nodded his head.

13

Research in palliative care nursing

Sheila Newman   Rosie Morton

INTRODUCTION

The very word 'research' creates a range of images that can include scientists in laboratories; academics in universities; or intense interviews to aid understanding. Whatever the context, neither author here believes that research needs to be dull or boring. Research enables both personal and professional development and, contrary to popular opinion, it also has the potential to be an interesting, engaging and even amusing journey of discovery.

Palliative care has three key features: it is a multidisciplinary specialty, based on humanistic values, and has a philosophy that strives for holistic care. This presents a broad and complex landscape to undertake the journey of research. Research journeys can follow many different paths but all should have a beginning, an end and a pathway that focus on the patient and those significant to them.

Caring for a person with an advanced incurable illness, whether it is cancer or non-malignant disease, and their loved ones and families, demands intelligence, creativity and compassion. Similar qualities are required in aiding research that engages interprofessional cooperation, and focuses on client perceptions as well as clinical need.

It has been strongly recommended that all nurses develop the ability to become critical readers and therefore discerning consumers of research (Department of Health 1993). The

personal and professional development. The value of research needs to be recognised and the values underpinning research studies need to be considered carefully if palliative care research is to have an impact on quality patient care.

As a relatively new specialty, in research terms, palliative care presents an opportunity for the development of research which harnesses multi-professional cooperation and focuses on client perceptions, as well as clinical need and evidence to support good practice.

Nurses have a critical role to play in meeting the challenge of initiating research that reflects the true nature of palliative care. Operationally and strategically, there is still much progress to be made. Palliative care nurses can and should exert significant influence in determining future agendas, leading research initiatives, ensuring collaboration with other professional groups and maximising dialogue, and the sharing of information, about research both formally and informally.

ACKNOWLEDGEMENT

Appreciation and thanks go to Phil Mackie and Alf Newman, for critical appraisal of a draft chapter.

REFERENCES

Addington-Hall J 1996 Heart disease and stroke, lessons from cancer care. In: Ford G, Lewin I (eds) Managing terminal illness. Royal College of Physicians, London

Ahmedzai S H 1997 Editorial: evidence-based medicine in palliative care: a systematic mistake? Progress in Palliative Care 5(3): 97–99

Aranda S 1995 Conducting research with the dying: ethical considerations and experience. International Journal of Palliative Nursing 1(1): 41–47

Armitage S 1990 Research utilisation in practice. Nurse Education Today 10: 10–15

Badger C 1994 Pause for thought: nurses use research don't they? European Journal of Cancer Care 3: 63–66

Benoliel J Q 1983 Nursing research on death, dying, and terminal illness: development, present state and prospects. Annual Review of Research 1: 101–130

Cawley N, Webber J 1995 Research priorities in palliative care. International Journal of Palliative Nursing 1(2): 101–113

Clark D 1997 What is qualitative research and what can it contribute to palliative care? Palliative Medicine 11: 159–166

Corner J 1996 Is there a research paradigm for palliative care? Palliative Medicine 10: 201–208

de Raeve L 1994 Ethical issues in palliative care research. Palliative Medicine 8: 298–305

Department of Health 1993 Report of the Taskforce on the Strategy for Research in Nursing, Midwifery and Health Visiting. Department of Health, London

Department of Health 1994 A Wider Strategy for Research And Development Relating to the Personal Social Services (The Smith Report). HMSO, London

Gibson V 1996 The problems of researching sensitive topics in health care. Nurse Researcher 4(2): 65–73

Glaser B G, Strauss A L 1965 Awareness of dying. Aldine, Chicago

Greenwood J 1984 Nursing research: a position paper. Journal of Advanced Nursing 9: 77–82

Hart E, Bond M 1996 Making sense of action research through the use of a typology. Journal of Advanced Nursing 23: 152–159

Hunt J 1981 Indicators for nursing practice: the use of research findings. Journal of Advanced Nursing 6: 189–194

Johnson B, Plant H 1996 In: de Raeve L (ed.) Nursing research an ethical and legal appraisal. Baillière Tindall, London

Keddy B, Sims S L, Stern P N 1996 Grounded theory as feminist research methodology. Journal of Advanced Nursing 23: 448–453

Kitzinger J 1995 Introducing focus groups. British Medical Journal 311: 299–302

Lorentzon M 1998 The way forward: nursing research or collaborative health care research? Journal of Advanced Nursing 27: 675–676

Macleod-Clark J, Hockey J 1989 Further research for nursing. Scutari Press, London

Morton R G 1995 Quality of life – what does this mean to patients who have oesophageal cancer? Unpublished research study

Mulhall A 1995 Nursing research: what difference does it make? Journal of Advanced Nursing 21: 576–583

NHS Executive 1998 A first class service: quality in the new NHS

Nolan M, Behi R 1995 What is research? Some definitions and dilemmas. British Journal of Nursing 4(2): 111–115

Payne S 1993 Constraints for nursing in developing a framework for cancer care research. European Journal of Cancer Care 2: 117–120

Pearcey P A 1995 Achieving research-based nursing practice. Journal of Advanced Nursing 22: 33–39

Pickering N 1996 In: de Raeve L (ed.) Nursing research an ethical and legal appraisal. Baillière Tindall, London

Reason P, Rowan J 1981 Human inquiry. John Wiley and Sons, Chichester

Richards M A, Corner J, Clark D 1998 Developing a research culture for palliative care. Palliative Medicine 12: 399–403

Richardson A, Wilson-Barnett J 1995 Nursing research in cancer care. Scutari Press, London

Rinck G C, van den Bos G A, Kleijnen J, de Haes H J, Schade E, Veenhof C H 1997 Methodologic issues in effectiveness research on palliative cancer care: a systematic review. Journal of Clinical Oncology 15(4): 1697–1707

Rolfe G 1994 Towards a new model of nursing research. Journal of Advanced Nursing 19: 969–975

Royal College of Nursing 1998 Clinical effectiveness. RCN, London

Royal College of Nursing 1995 A guide to planning our career. RCN, London

Seymour J, Clark D 1998 Phenomenological approach to palliative care research. Palliative Medicine 12: 127–131

Seymour J E, Ingleton C 1999 Ethical issues in qualitative research at the end of life. International Journal of Palliative Nursing 5(2): 65–73

Walters A J 1995 The phenomenological movement: implications for nursing research. Journal of Advanced Nursing 22: 791–799

Wilkes 1998 Palliative care nursing research: trends from 1987 to 1996. International Journal of Palliative Nursing 4(3): 128–134

Wilson-Barnett J, Richardson A 1998 In: Doyle D, Hanks G W C, MacDonald N (eds) Oxford textbook of palliative medicine. Oxford Medical Publications, Oxford

FURTHER READING

Beaver K, Luker K, Woods S 1999 Conducting research with the terminally ill: challenges and considerations. International Journal of Palliative Nursing 5(1): 13–17

Behi R, Nolan M 1995 Ethical issues in research. British Journal of Nursing 4(12): 712–716

Britten N 1995 Qualitative interviews in medical research. British Medical Journal 311: 251–253

Corner J 1991 In search of more complete answers to research questions. Quantitative versus qualitative research methods: is there a way forward? Journal of Advanced Nursing 16: 718–727

Corner J 1991 Cancer nursing research. Nursing Times 87(37): 42–44

Corner J 1993 Building a framework for nursing research in cancer care. European Journal of Cancer Care 2: 112–116

Cowles K V 1988 Issues in qualitative research on sensitive topics. Western Journal of Nursing Research 10(2): 163–179

Crowther T, Biswas B, Randall F, Macpherson D, Wells F 1994 Guidelines on Research in Palliative Care. The National Council for Hospices and Specialist Palliative Care Services

Doyle D 1993 Editorial – palliative medicine – a time for definition? Palliative Medicine 7: 253–255

Duley L 1996 Systematic reviews: what can they do for you? Journal of the Royal Society of Medicine 89: 242–244

Faithfull S 1996 How many subjects are needed in a research sample in palliative care? Palliative Medicine 10: 259–261

Ford G 1994 Definition and prospects. Palliative Care Today 3(11): 21

Hagemaster J N 1992 Life history: a qualitative method of research. Journal of Advanced Nursing 17: 1122–1128

Hanson E J 1994 Issues concerning the familiarity of researchers with the research setting. Journal of Advanced Nursing 20: 940–942

Ingleton C, Field D, Clark D 1998 Formative evaluation and its relevance to palliative care. Palliative Medicine 12: 197–203

International Council of Nurses 1996 Better health through nursing research. ICN, Geneva

Jones J, Hunter D 1995 Consensus methods for medical and health services research. British Medical Journal 311: 376–380

Keen J, Packwood T 1995 Case study evaluation. British Medical Journal 311: 444–446

Lelean S R, Clarke M 1990 Research resource development in the United Kingdom. International Journal of Nursing Studies 27(2): 123–138

Ling J, Penn K 1995 The challenges of conducting clinical trials in palliative care. International Journal of Palliative Nursing 1(1): 31–34

Lowden B 1998 Introducing palliative care: health professionals' perceptions. International Journal of Palliative Nursing 4(3): 135–142

May K A 1979 The nurse as researcher: impediment to informed consent? Nursing Outlook 36–39

Mays N, Pope C 1995 Rigour and qualitative research. British Medical Journal 311: 109–112

Meyer J E 1993 New paradigm research in practice: the trials and tribulations of action research. Journal of Advanced Nursing 18: 1066–1072

Mirolo B, Bunce I H, Chapman M et al 1995 Psychosocial benefits of postmastectomy lymphoedema therapy. Cancer Nursing 18(3): 197–205

Nolan M, Behi R 1995 Research in nursing: developing a conceptual approach. British Journal of Nursing 4(1): 47–50

Nolan M, Behi R 1995 Alternative approaches to establishing reliability and validity. British Journal of Nursing 4(10): 587–590

Oleske D M, Heinze S, Otte D M 1990 The diary as a means of understanding the quality of life of persons with cancer receiving home nursing care. Cancer Nursing 13(3): 158–166

Payne S 1997 Selecting an approach and design in qualitative research. Palliative Medicine 11: 249–252

Plant H 1996 Research interviewing. Palliative Medicine 10: 339–341

Pope C, Mays N 1995 Reaching the parts other methods cannot reach: an introduction to qualitative methods in health and health services research. British Medical Journal 311: 42–45

Royal College of Nursing 1998 Research Ethics. RCN, London

Scullion J E, Henry C 1998 A multidisciplinary approach to managing breathlessness in lung cancer. International Journal of Palliative Nursing 4(2): 65–69

to issues and by reflecting on both personal values and the ethical principles involved in the issue, the reader should be able to objectively examine the ethical permissibility of clinical actions within palliative health care. Far from ethics being a dry subject, it is anticipated that the reader will be drawn into constructive, informed critical argument and debate, bringing alive the ethics within palliative care.

THE MORAL PICTURE

The provision of health care is becoming increasingly complicated by the expectations of a society which is better informed about current treatment options and has high demands and high expectations about the health care provided. The focus of palliative care, by its very definition, looks towards multi-professional holistic care provision following recognition of no potential cure. This places an emphasis upon individual preferences in determining the quality of life. The subjective issues that arise should be considered on an individual basis, and should be recognised as reflecting values that are the essence of individualised care. In attempting to provide appropriate care, health care professionals may find conflict between their assessment of the needs of the patient and their family, the interventions deemed necessary by both parties, and in determining objectively the general subjective priorities that individuals place on their own value and quality of life.

In general, ethics can only provide an indication of the general ethical permissibility or acceptability of actions. If carers respect even the most fundamental principles of ethics, the autonomy of the individual patient should be respected; this is balanced by the principles of beneficence and non-maleficence. However, decisions that are arrived at result in implications for our society in general and, as such, the ethical permissibility of care for individuals needs to be tapered by the implications for the ethical implications of similar situations within our society – the notion of the principle of justice.

Ethical issues that arise in palliative care may be recognised as being similar to those in other specialties. Common examples include issues affecting the professional–patient relationship, resource allocation, truth-telling, confidentiality, respect of individual and professional autonomy, consent to and refusal of treatment and the withholding and the withdrawal of treatments at both the macro- and micro-level within palliative care.

All too frequently palliative ethics is mistakenly focused on the debate surrounding euthanasia. The reality is that the nature of the very concept of palliative care, particularly within the hospice network, excludes the euthanasia debate in that palliative care by its very definition does *not* intentionally hasten, shorten or unnecessarily prolong the end of life of those in receipt of quality palliative care. Palliative care cannot therefore include the deliberate ending of life within its objectives, whether it is actively or passively sought, either voluntarily or non-voluntarily.

Palliative care continues to be challenged in recognising the extent and alleviating the spiritual, psychological and social symptoms in addition to the ongoing relief of physical needs. Regrettably, at times, carers and families become the reluctant observers of inadequate symptom control, where suffering, distress and fear become unmanageable by the multi-professional team. At these times it is possible to begin to understand the view of some who place such value on their lives not to wish to experience such distress, and would prefer to shorten their natural lives. This brings up the emotive subject of passive voluntary euthanasia.

Reflection point

From the issues already identified:

- Can you recognise instances in your professional career where you were faced with a professional dilemma about one or more of these issues?
- How did you come to the decision you made?
- What influenced you at that point in time?
- On reflection would you make the same decisions now?
- If not, then what circumstances might influence your current values?
- If you had to make similar decisions outside of your professional life, would your decisions reflect similar outcomes to your professional decisions?

ETHICAL ISSUES IN PALLIATIVE CARE

While these issues may be similar to those experienced in other health specialties there exists a unique edge to some ethical dilemmas in the specialty of palliative care. The very nature of palliative care focuses debate about ethical issues on the inevitable death of the person. Circumstances at the end of life may result in ethical dilemmas being further complicated by issues concerning the competence of the dying person, their right to refuse or accept care and in maintaining their personal integrity over their own death. Ethical dilemmas may arise from differing values placed upon the value of life by both patients and their carers. Dilemmas may also extend to circumstances surrounding resource distribution: do dying people have the right to access every possible treatment whatever the cost in terms of finance, time and available resources? It would appear that palliative care has a unique set of ethical situations that challenge the multi-professional team, the patient and their families to determine ethically permissible courses of action.

In bringing comfort and hope to patients and their families who are in need of quality palliative care, multi-professional health care teams are frequently challenged by decisions that need to be made depending on the circumstances at a particular time. Potential influences on these decisions can be seen in Box 14.1.

Box 14.1 Potential influences on ethical decision making

- Law
- Professional codes of conduct
- Societal and cultural values
- Personal values and beliefs

The influence of the laws of individual states on ethical decisions determine the legal rightness or wrongness of actions, not necessarily their moral ethical permissibility. This situation is clearly illustrated by the issue of assisted suicide where the law determines the legality of such actions (whether the action or omission is ethically permissible or not). This is illustrated by assisted suicide being currently illegal in the UK; a very grey area in Holland (being non-legalised, but not appearing to be legally punished by society); being legalised and then overturned in the Northern Territories in Australia during the late 1990s; and being legal (given specific circumstances) in the state of Oregon in the United States where one can apply to have a prescription for medication to end one's life (the safeguards of this are controlled through strict criteria including a 'cooling off' period in case the subject changes their mind!).

Those who work in palliative care may understand the wishes of patients who wish to die peacefully and with a quality of life whose acceptability can only be determined by the patient themselves. In some situations patients may *value* an early *end to their lives*. While perhaps not agreeing with some practices, it is a compassion of understanding that health care professionals are required to develop in such circumstances, respecting the autonomy of the individual's wishes.

For a simple example of an ethical dilemma in palliative care consider the concerns about truth-telling. Consider the *hypothetical* scenario shown in Case study 14.1.

Consideration of ethics may not provide the answer to all the difficult questions that can arise in palliative care. Frequently, there is no clear right or wrong, black or white side to a clinical situation, only a greyish state of affairs that appears to change depending on the way the overall picture is perceived.

What ethics does allow for is specific argument to be made about the circumstances surrounding individual cases which looks to answer the question, not of whether the result is essentially right or wrong, but whether it is *ethically permissible*. In ethics the emphasis must be regarded and thought of in terms of the ethical permissibility of actions or inactions. An awareness of ethical issues and arguments enables practitioners to come to informed decisions about their actions and to help clarify situations for patients and their families.

The challenges faced by health care professionals within palliative care are frequently focused around specific ethical issues at the end of life (Fig. 14.1), such as decisions relating to the continued provision of artificial hydration, certain drugs and artificial feeding. These are in addition to the general issues that commonly affect most clinical specialties as well as palliative care. Ethics can provide a basis to determine whether decisions made about care, treatments or withholding treatments can be ethically permissible.

Decisions are complicated further when a patient's personal autonomy is reduced. This can occur when the patient may no longer be able to indicate their personal preference as a result of drugs, a progressive deterioration of their consciousness or through any disease process that restricts their ability to understand, to deliberate or to communicate their wishes (or any combination of these). In such circumstances, consideration of actions that would be in the best interests of the patient need to be determined. This can be facilitated through discussion with close family members or, in their absence, the multi-professional team providing the care. Difficulties can arise through conflict amongst immediate family or team members when, as individual people, they have differing values about issues at the end of life.

Even during the provision of palliative care during the early stages of a disease process there are difficult decisions to be made about the provision of expensive treatments. Such resource allocations are not just linked to individual treatments but to the decisions made by Trusts and Health Management Executives about the provision of

certain long-term treatments (e.g. a particular drug treatment available for patients with multiple sclerosis which may not be available in all parts of the country). Equally, the preferences of patients to die within their home environment may be restricted by the local availability of appropriate care in the community, or the availability of local palliative units within remote rural areas, which necessitates family members having to travel large distance at a time when they may be increasingly vulnerable.

The Calman–Hine (1995) report went some way to recognising the need to achieve equality in the availability and provision of cancer care and, as a consequence, palliative care across the country. Such initiatives are to be applauded, but must be continually acted upon to maximise the benefit to patients who require palliative care regardless of the nature of the cause.

The ethics around euthanasia can be debated from many angles, both for and against. Individuals need to decide what they feel is ethically appropriate. However, while defending the right of individuals to self-determination, it may not be ethically appropriate to request that someone assists in the death of a person if they are not willing to do so, or if it challenges the professional code in which they work, or if it challenges the legal circumstances in that country. The concept of euthanasia takes many forms: voluntary or nonvoluntary, passive or active. In Utopia, all symp-

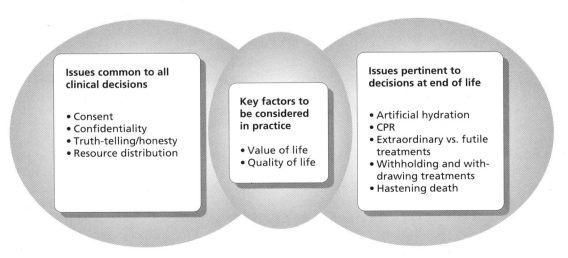

Figure 14.1   Ethical issues in palliative care.

toms in palliative care could be addressed, not just the physical but the psychological, social and spiritual. In reality, health care is only able to meet some of these admirable goals; but in striving for them practitioners should never lose sight of the individual patient and his/her family. Guidelines from The National Council for Hospice and Specialist Palliative Care Services (NCHSPCS) focus on the non-acceptance of voluntary euthanasia (NCHSPCS 1992, 1997a). These guidelines should be adhered to by those involved in palliative care; however, practitioners should be aware of the ethical arguments that underpin both sides of this emotive issue, and, as the NCHSPCS guidelines do, *recognise the right of the individual to request* to be allowed to hasten death, or to refuse treatment that results in the hastening of death.

ETHICAL THEORIES

Two differing but highly influential ethical theories have influenced the morals of current society. Together with key ethical principles that influence current health care provision, these factors form the basis on which the ethical permissibility of clinical decisions across health care, and in particular palliative care, are based. An ethical approach to determining whether actions or inactions are ethically permissible, which includes consideration about the quality and the value of life and death, should in turn bring comfort and hope to patients and their families.

In considering clinical decisions or dilemmas there are several ethical approaches that can be used. The two key theoretical approaches that are introduced in this chapter reflect a duty-based approach – deontology, and a consequence-based approach – consequentialism.

Deontology

Approaches that involve basing decisions according to a duty that follows certain rules which should always be adhered to, whatever the circumstances, are known as *deontological* approaches. These approaches resolving ethical dilemmas stem from the work of Kant, and rely upon individuals adhering to specific 'rules'.

Actions or inactions are considered to be ethically unacceptable if these are contravened. Kant refers to these 'rules' as categorical imperatives which must apply in all situations – they are universal. These include 'rules' of not killing and of telling the truth. Problems for deontological approaches to health care arise when the truth can cause harm to the patient or their family or in providing treatment that might have a foreseeable side-effect of harming or ending the life of a patient.

Consequentialism

Alternatively, decisions may be based on the potential consequences of one's actions, which is consequentialism. Consequence-based ethical approaches are concerned solely on making decisions depending on the consequences that occur from the actions of the decision. Consequentialist approaches to ethics have developed from the utilitarian theories of Mill and Bentham. Their aim is that actions or inactions are ethically permissible where they maximise benefit or minimise harm as a consequence. As such, certain actions may become ethically permissible even if it means that certain 'rules' have to be broken. For example, a consequentialist could argue that it is ethically permissible to hasten the end of the life of a person if the consequences of that action would be to maximise the benefit for the person involved and perhaps for many others. There are two types of utilitarians: act utilitarians and rule utilitarians. The former would always act by considering the good and bad consequences in each particular set of circumstances; the latter would resolve to follow actions based on determining the consequences in similar circumstances.

While consequentialist approaches to decision making can appear advantageous to some, the difficulty with determining the ethical permissibility lies in the determination of what constitutes 'happiness and harm'. For some people happiness may be derived from harm. The actual measure of the amount of 'happiness' may cause difficulty in determining the overall consequence of our actions. What may maximise benefit to one person may only be a minor happiness to

15

The disadvantaged dying – care of people with non-malignant conditions

Michael J. Connolly

INTRODUCTION

Palliative care challenges the medical model of health care. A doctor-driven agenda may possibly be justified in curative care but there is a need for a patient-centred and multidisciplinary approach with those we cannot cure. Corner (1997) describes nurses as having become analogous to flight attendants in health care, taking pride in the diligent and humane obedience to the medical world. Nursing has almost always worked in a supplementary and, sometimes, complementary role to medicine; only occasionally has a stronger role been found for nurses and the professions allied to medicine (PAMs).

Corner suggests that nursing should reject this role, be careful of accumulating the tedious and peripheral tasks of junior doctors and claim its own position as an autonomous, research-based and confident profession. The challenge is there, both for nursing and for palliative care. Whenever science-based, technical medicine runs out of answers, whenever, after the best efforts of modern medicine, the patient is left with a range of interconnected problems, few solutions and considerable distress, then a different approach is needed. This is where palliative care has built its movement. This chapter describes what palliative care has done for people with cancer and what it must also do for those living and dying with non-malignant diseases. The chapter argues that it is logical to expect nurses to lead the way with this new challenge and that, in doing so, nurses can help focus nursing onto what it does best. The research evidence is not extensive and therefore the arguments are supported by what research there is, by the conclusions of a recent national working party (Addington-Hall 1998) and by the clinical experiences of the author.

Palliative care asks for a paradigm shift, a change in the way that the situation is looked at: a shift from disease management to personal support and care which may, at times, involve symptom and disease management. This is not to replace the medical or disease management model with a nursing-dominated model but to allow a patient-focused model to emerge. The change of perspective attempts to view the symptoms and problems through patients' eyes: it tries to understand their agenda. Once seen in this light, it becomes inconceivable to fail to involve patients in decision making or to tell them that 'there is nothing more to be done', to see communication skills as merely added value, unnecessary icing on the cake of medical, diagnostic expertise. This model is, or should be, 'home territory' for nursing.

Palliative care represents, therefore, a challenge to the medical orthodoxy. The shift in perspective is likely to be most easily understood in primary care, elderly care, in therapies allied to medicine and in nursing. The corollary is that the challenge of palliative care is likely to be most difficult for doctors, particularly those in hospital medicine, where the 'acute', disease management model is strongest.

A junior doctor recently described to me the case of a man he had seen in Accident and Emergency. The man, who had advanced cancer, was unable to swallow, was semiconscious and was in some distress. His daughter was upset that she had been unable to care for him at home but she was furious that her father was being actively revived in the hospital. The doctor explained his position to me: 'It's clear to me, that since his haemoglobin was 6.5, I had a moral and ethical duty to transfuse four units of blood'. It was clear to me that the pathology was being managed but the patient and his family were being ignored. My task was to help pacify his angry relatives and to engage in a debate with the doctor about his ethical and legal position.

These purposes of palliative care and the roles for nursing within it are presented as a backdrop or foundation for the main focus of this chapter, i.e. non-malignant disease.

NON-MALIGNANT DISEASE

The man with nausea and vomiting, urinary problems, isolation and weakness has cor pulmonale. Like 75% of those who die, he does not have cancer. This makes him one of the disadvantaged dying.
(Dobratz 1990)

A hugely influential and still relevant study (Hinton 1963) found that the amount of physical distress associated with heart failure and renal failure was greater than that experienced by people with cancer. Pain was the exception to these findings, with a higher incidence in cancer. More recent studies suggest that people with cancer report more and more distressing symptoms, particularly pain, in the last months of life (Seale 1991, Addington-Hall 1996, Addington-Hall et al 1998).

Cerebrovascular disease accounts for 12% of all deaths; there is little literature on the care received by those who die of stroke. A British study (Addington-Hall et al 1995), 'The Regional Study of the Care of the Dying', found that in the last week of life, stroke patients experienced urinary incontinence (51%), pain (42%), mental confusion (41%), low mood (33%) and faecal incontinence (31%). The authors of this study conclude that: 'because it is difficult to make accurate judgments about symptoms experienced by patients whose ability to communicate has been affected by stroke, these results may underestimate the misery caused by poorly controlled symptoms'.

A large American study 'The Study to Understand Prognoses and Preferences for Outcomes and Risks of Treatments (SUPPORT)' (Lynn et al 1997b) which is in some ways similar to the British studies mentioned above (it interviewed close relatives after the patient had died), provides an insight into the relationship between the care that people want and the care they receive. Of 3357 patients who had died, 4 in 10 had severe pain in the last 3 days of life, 55% were conscious, severe fatigue affected almost 8 in 10 patients and 63% had difficulty tolerating physical or emotional symptoms. Overall, 11% had a final resuscitation attempt. A ventilator was used in one-quarter of patients and a feeding tube was used in 40% of patients. Most patients (59%) were reported to prefer a treatment plan that focused on comfort, but care was reported to be contrary to the preferred approach in 10% of cases (Figs 15.1 and 15.2).

Diagnosing dying

The SUPPORT study evidence suggests that the disease is being managed right up to the point of death and the symptoms are commonly not well controlled. The reasons for this are likely to be several and complicated. One such reason seems to be that health professionals find it difficult to diagnose dying. A study looking at the predicted life expectancy of patients who actually died the next day confirms anecdotal evidence that death in non-malignant conditions is harder to predict than it is in cancer.

Lynn et al (1997a) describe the results of two major studies in the United States which show that:

One often cannot rely upon there being a period of time in which dying is evidently near which is also long enough to allow those involved to embark upon planning for death.

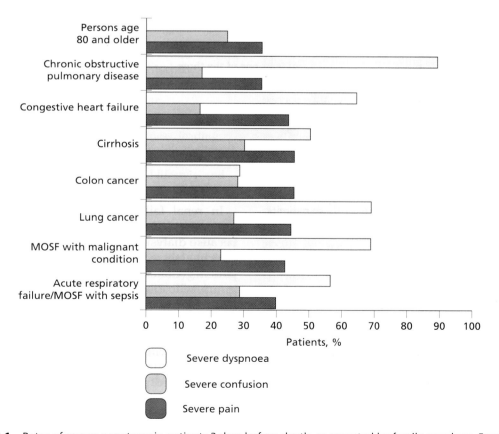

Figure 15.1 Rates of severe symptoms in patients 3 days before death, as reported by family members. Family members of elderly patients were not asked about dyspnoea. MOSF, multiple organ system failure. From Lynn et al 1997b, with permission.

WHAT ARE THE DIFFICULTIES OF DEVELOPING PALLIATIVE CARE IN THIS WAY?

There are good reasons why specialist palliative care services should be wary of opening up their services to people with non-malignant diseases:

- existing services will be overwhelmed
- the disease trajectory is difficult to determine; estimates of time to death are too inaccurate
- Will the specialists in palliative care have the expertise?
- Will there be extra resources to allow this development?
- Will cancer patients be neglected?

Higginson (1995) has led the field in her work to establish some way of estimating the need for palliative care services. Her epidemiological approach has looked at the prevalence of cancer, the demand for palliative care services and the prevalence of other diseases, that in terms of symptoms and prognosis are comparable with cancer.

Her estimation is that there is likely to be as much need in non-malignant disease as there is in cancer. We know that the palliative care services for people with cancer are not uniformly good, complete or accessible. It is an irony that while providers of palliative care insist to health planners that the palliative care services for people with cancer are unequal and underfunded, the health planners then ask the providers to double their workload.

WHAT ARE THE DRIVING FORCES?

The political pressure to define palliative care in a way that includes non-malignant disease has become irresistible. The principal argument is one of equity. How can health planners and commissioners justify spending money on palliative care services for only about a half of those who are likely to need them? However, the existing palliative care services are only partly paid for from public money, normally considerably less than half the real costs. Torrens (1981) warned that 'the independent hospices have been able to develop freely . . . the cost of more secure fund-

ing may well be greater regulation'. There are some in the hospice movement who feel that there is much greater regulation without necessarily more secure funding. There is a debate within specialist palliative care as to whether it is reasonable to ask them to provide services on an equal footing to the cancer-based services to the people with non-malignant disease. The Department of Health is clear about its intentions:

All patients needing them should have access to palliative care services. Although often referred to as equating with terminal care, it is important to recognise that similar services are appropriate and should be developed for patients dying from other diseases.   (SMAC SNMAC 1992)

Purchasers are asked to ensure that provision of palliative care with a palliative approach is included in all contracts of service for those with cancer and other life threatening diseases . . . although this letter is focussed on services for cancer patients, it applies equally for patients with other life threatening conditions, including AIDS, neurological conditions, and cardiac and respiratory failure.
(NHS Executive 1996)

A number of surveys have shown that general practitioners would welcome access to and advice from specialist palliative care services for patients with non-malignant disease (Kurti & O'Dowd 1995, Wilson et al 1995). Apart from GPs, however, there is little to suggest any great call from health workers in non-malignant disease for palliative care specialists to help them with their patients. Equally, there is no great appetite to vastly widen the remit of palliative care from within the movement itself, so it is clear that the major drivers for this change emanate from political circles and, more recently, from the NCHSPCS.

It is important to note that before the modern hospice world began to focus upon people with cancer, that there were no advantaged dying groups. Palliative care has not consciously neglected non-malignant disease; it has simply concentrated on one of the most feared illnesses of modern times – cancer. Addington-Hall (1998) suggests that the work is far from done in cancer care:

Despite the growth in hospice and specialist palliative care services, population based studies have shown that some cancer patients are still receiving inadequate care, and have unmet needs for symptom control and psychological support.

Specialist palliative care services in the UK have overwhelmingly catered for people with cancer. The NCHSPCS report suggests that, from a sample of palliative care teams, the proportion of patients who did not have cancer in the workloads of those teams was between 0% and 12%, with a median of 5%. The working party concluded that specialist palliative care provision to people with non-malignant disease is likely to be highest in the hospitals but that, even there, they are seeing people with cancer 95% of the time, despite cancer only representing 25% of deaths.

> **Reflection point**
>
> How can palliative care services adapt to become more relevant/accessible to people with non-malignant diseases?

DOES PALLIATIVE CARE HAVE THE RESOURCES TO HELP?

This chapter has described two of the frontiers of palliative care, namely non-malignant disease and the acute hospital sector; there is at least one other frontier which the movement has been exploring for some years. This third frontier is the move to apply palliative care principles and services to the needs of people at earlier stages of their illness.

We have learned a great deal about the needs of people with cancer, more particularly we have learned a great deal about people who are dying of cancer; we have chosen a very specific group of people to work with.   (Torrens 1981)

Any army fighting on too many fronts is vulnerable. To spread ourselves too thinly and too quickly at such an early stage in the history of our movement, may turn out to be a tactical mistake. If we are to work in hospitals, with non-malignant disease and from diagnosis to death, are we risking a return to the neglect of the dying cancer patient?

We must ask ourselves whether we are sufficiently confident with our aims, our values and our expertise. The next question is about whether we have the soldiers to fight on so many fronts.

The answer to this latter question is possibly to be found amongst nurses in palliative care and in non-malignant disease.

As the palliative care movement considers its role in non-malignant disease, it must be mindful that there is still much to be done within palliative care in cancer care to fully establish the role and position of nursing and to place patients rather than illness as the prime concern.

It is the developments within palliative care nursing, the range of influences that nursing has had within palliative care, that provide some of the guides/clues as to how palliative care as a movement could make an impact in renal failure, COAD, stroke, heart failure, etc.

> **Reflection point**
>
> Who has the responsibility to bring the advantages of the palliative care approach and specialist palliative care to people with non-malignant diseases?
>
> - Nurses and others on palliative care
> - Nurses and others on cardiology, respiratory medicine, renal medicine, etc.
> - Nurses and others in primary care
> - Health planners

THE ROLE OF NURSING AND OF NURSES

The clinical nurse specialist role in cancer and palliative care has been pioneered by Macmillan Cancer Relief; this has been a contribution to the profession of nursing, as in this field these nurses have often spearheaded the frontiers of the movement. By and large the move out of hospices was led by community-based clinical nurse specialists in palliative care (Macmillan nurses); the same has been the case within the general hospital sector – nurse specialists first, followed by consultants some years later.

This pattern should give nurses the confidence of their own success and should guide plans when considering palliative care in non-malignant disease. Nurses could lead at this new frontier and the voluntary and charitable sector may well be the engine that powers the movement.

The NCHSPCS report refers specifically to clinical nurse specialist posts as one clear way forward:

There are already clinical nurse specialists who specialise in, for example, respiratory disease, rheumatoid arthritis and Parkinson's disease. These nurses . . . play an important role in patient and family support and have specific expertise in the management of the disease. An increase in funding for these posts, together with educational programmes to enable these valuable specialist nurses to adopt confidently the palliative care approach in addition to their existing skills, and the development of professional links with specialist palliative care teams, may be one way to improve the palliative care received by patients with non-malignant disease.

The equivalent in the community may be the development of more link nurse posts: community nurses with extra training in palliative care, who provide a link between the community nurse colleagues and clinical nurse specialists in palliative care posts is a possibility, provided that they are part of specialist palliative care teams.

A major advantage of this would be that nurses would be able to develop disease specific expertise, but the potential for further fragmentation needs to be considered.

THE ROLE OF THE VOLUNTARY SECTOR IN PALLIATIVE CARE

The partnership between the NHS and the voluntary sector is now strong in the cancer services.

It is likely, but regrettable, that palliative care services will have to continue to be largely funded by the local and national charities. I believe that this perpetuates the impression that palliative care is in some way an added extra – the icing on the cake. Not only does this impression leave palliative care services open to financial cutting but it leaves doubt in the minds of health professionals as to the real value of the care. It is for these reasons that the palliative care movement needs at the same time to be compassionate and humane while also being evidence-based and scientific.

There is another argument, however; the partnership between the NHS and the voluntary sector could become a model for other fields of health care. I suggest that it may be the right model for the move to include people with non-malignant disease in palliative care provision. The voluntary sector (mostly the independent hospices, with the significant addition of the major cancer charities) has enabled the palliative care movement to be innovative in practice, research and teaching; it has paid for new posts in the heart of NHS provision years before the NHS services were sure that they should spend money on palliative care. And it has maintained a relationship with its donors that has captured the imagination of the public. The voluntary sector is likely to continue to be the driving force behind palliative care in all areas.

CONCLUSION

The proposed extension of palliative care to non-malignant disease, and the arrival of non-malignant disease to palliative care, presents a challenge and an opportunity to palliative care and to nurses in particular. There is a need for palliative care expertise within the care of people with non-malignant disease. It is not clear exactly what help is most appropriate or what help will be welcomed. It does seem clear, however, that there are enough similarities between the needs of cancer patients and those of other patients with life-threatening illnesses for the links between palliative care and non-malignant disease to be explored. The palliative care movement has a short history that is characterised by innovation, statutory and voluntary sector collaboration and by nurses as change agents. It seems likely that with tact, humility, a desire to understand and some determination, the boundaries can be dismantled and the clear benefits that effective palliative care can bring can be brought to the 'disadvantaged dying'.

REFERENCES

Addington-Hall J 1996 Heart disease and stroke: lessons from cancer care. In: Ford G, Lewin I (eds) Interfaces in medicine: managing terminal illness. Royal College of Physicians, London

Addington-Hall J 1998 Reaching out: specialist palliative care for adults with non-malignant disease. National Council for Hospices and Specialist Palliative Care Services, London

Addington-Hall J M, Lay M, Altman D, McCarthy M 1995 Symptom control, communication with health professionals and hospital care of stroke patients in the last year of life, as reported by surviving family, friends and carers. Stroke 26: 2242–2248

Addington-Hall J, Altman D, McCarthy M 1998 Variations in age in symptoms and dependency levels experienced by people in the last year of life, as reported by surviving family, friends and officials. Age and Ageing 27: 129–136

Cohen L M, McCue J D, Germain M, Kjellstrand C M 1995 Dialysis discontinuation. A 'good' death? Archives of Internal Medicine 155: 42–47

Corner J 1997 Nursing and the counter culture for cancer. European Journal of Cancer Care 6: 174–181

Dobratz M C 1990 Hospice nursing: present perspectives and future directions. Cancer Nursing 13: 116–122

Gibson J, Kenrick M 1998 Pain and powerlessness: the experience of living with peripheral vascular disease. Journal of Advanced Nursing 27: 737–745

Hearn J, Higginson I 1998 Do specialist palliative care teams improve outcomes for cancer patients? A systematic literature review. Palliative Medicine 12: 317–332

Higginson I J 1995 Epidemiologically-based needs assessment for palliative and terminal care. NHS Executive, Leeds

Hinton J M 1963 The physical and mental distress of the dying. Quarterly Medical Journal 32: 1–21

Kurti L G, O'Dowd T C 1995 Dying of non-malignant diseases in general practice. Journal of Palliative Care 11: 25–31

Lynn J, Harrell F, Cohn F, Wagner D, Connors A 1997a Prognoses of seriously ill hospitalised patients on the days before death: implications for patient care and public policy. New Horizons 5: 56–61

Lynn J, Teno J M, Philips R S et al 1997b Perceptions by family members of the dying experience of older and seriously ill patients. Annals of Internal Medicine 126: 97–106

NHS Executive 1996 A policy framework for commissioning cancer services: palliative care services. EL(96)85. NHS Executive, London

Salisbury C, Bosanquet N, Wilkinson E K et al 1999 the impact of different models of specialist palliative care on patient's quality of life: a systematic literature review. Palliative Medicine 13: 3–17

Seale C 1991 Death from cancer and death from other causes: the relevance of the hospice approach. Palliative Medicine 5: 13–20

Skillbeck J, Mott L, Page H, Smith D, Ahmedzai S, Clark D 1998 Palliative care in chronic obstructive airways disease: a needs assessment. Palliative Medicine 12: 245–254

Standing Medical Advisory Committee (SMAC), Standing Nursing and Midwifery Committee (SNMC) 1992 The principles and provision of palliative care. Department of Health, London

Torrens P 1981 Achievements, failure and the future of hospice. In: Saunders C (ed.) Hospice the living idea. Arnold, London

Wilson I M, Bunting J S, Curnow R M, Knock J 1995 The need for inpatient palliative care facilities for non-cancer patients in Thames Valley. Palliative Medicine 9: 13–18

Fallowfield (1990) believes we are entering an ethically challenging period in modern medicine when QOL issues must be considered. Because it is now possible to keep alive patients who would have previously died, the use of new technologies must be questioned. New anticancer drugs are usually tested on patients with advanced cancer in the final phase of their trials. Although patients willingly enter into such trials, even though they are informed that cure is no longer an option for them, one wonders if they realise how much more miserable their final days may be due to the side effects of the drugs. Research seems to indicate that younger patients and, understandably, those with a partner or children are more likely to accept chemotherapy even when there is an insignificant possibility of improvement (Bremnes et al 1995).

When chemotherapy is considered for patients with advanced cancer, the decision for or against treatment must be based on the probability that palliation will be achieved: that chemotherapy will improve QOL can be difficult to predict. The effect of chemotherapy on QOL is or should be a major factor influencing treatment choice.

'Quality of life' is a conceptual model, intended to represent the perspective of the patient in quantifiable terms. According to Cella (1992) there are two fundamental components of QOL: subjectivity and multidimensionality. Subjectivity refers to the fact that QOL can only be determined by the patient, and only by asking the patient directly can the subjective component be assessed.

Defining QOL can be problematic. The politician, the philosopher, the priest, the psychologist, the physician and the patient would all offer different definitions; it can difficult to measure what we cannot clearly define.

Dudgeon (1992) identifies that conflict between nurses and physicians frequently centres around QOL issues. One of the reasons suggested for this conflict originates in part from the different models of practice used by doctors and nurses. Traditional Western medicine is based on the biomedical disease model, which is reductionist in nature; man is reduced to a number of inter-related parts. This model of man tends to be mechanistic in its approach in that parts can be removed and replaced when required. Outcomes are sought which are observable, measurable and predictable. Survival rates and physical function are measurable; therefore, they have proved useful measures of outcome.

Dudgeon goes on to suggest that the biomedical model leaves little or no room for the psychological, social, behavioural and spiritual dimensions. Nursing, while strongly influenced by the biomedical model, has rejected the reductionist mind–body dualism of the full version of this model (Feil & Hahn Winslow 1985).

There are many nursing models in current use, most of which claim to be holistic in nature. Nurses appear to be concerned with psychosocial issues. Dudgeon (1992) studied the entries in patient case notes made by doctors and nurses, noting that nurses documented emotional issues and family relationships 2.5 times more than doctors did. It was noted that nurses paid attention to non-biological issues; such issues contribute to QOL. Dudgeon suggests that a QOL model should be used by both doctors and nurses evaluating the effect of disease and, together with medical and psychosocial interventions, could bring the biomedical and the nursing model closer together. If improvement in QOL becomes the diagnostic and therapeutic goal, conflict between nurses and doctors would be reduced. Dudgeon (1992) goes on to propose that the use of a QOL model could provide the bridge between medicine and nursing. This view, however, fails to acknowledge that doctors and nurses may continue to have different ideas about what QOL is.

Schipper (1992) points out that medicine is highly culture-dependent. Models of disease and medicine are inextricably rooted in their host culture. What is viewed as an illness in one culture may not be considered an illness in another. Treatments that are acceptable in one culture, may not be accepted in another. Illness has a different meaning for each observer of the process: for the nurse caregiver, it means suffering to be relieved; for the family, it means changes in relationships; for the patient, it represents a threat to well-being, longevity and expectation. Each observer has a particular culture-dependent model that is applied to the process.

Both doctors and nurses are poor at assessing patient QOL according to Slevin et al (1988).

'Quality of life' is a conceptual model intended to represent the perspective of the patient in quantifiable terms. In this way, QOL can be viewed as a final common pathway measure that represents the net effect of the disease and all the medical and psychosocial therapies. Schipper (1992) suggests that if the QOL model is understood and valued by all parties it provides a common language.

HOW MIGHT WE DEFINE QUALITY OF LIFE?

QOL is an abstract idea, not bound by time or place; it is situational and encompasses many overlapping concepts (Mast 1995). The philosopher Brock (1993) considers QOL to have three main theoretical considerations:

1. The human condition described in terms of feelings of happiness and satisfaction or lack of the same.
2. The capabilities of the human being in terms of function and performance, which may include role function; this is age-related.
3. The preference satisfaction theory, which includes complex issues such as choice, freedom of access and patient autonomy.

Culture and country of residence will influence the third consideration. Calman (1984) proposed an integration of these, and suggested that 'quality of life' measures the difference, at a particular moment in time, between the hopes and expectations of an individual and that individual's present experiences. Hence, just as values may differ according to age group, expectations regarding QOL will also differ according to age and stage in the life cycle (Berado 1992). The family life stages of the patient and caregiver are connected to their psychosocial adjustment to illness. Indeed, many would argue that we couldn't consider the quality of life of an individual without considering that of the caregiver (Parker 1990, Biegel et al 1991). It is broadly accepted conventional wisdom that care in the community is better than

institutional care. However, the care of one family member may place an undue burden on another. To maintain the QOL of one person may decrease that of another. Cella (1992) identifies that extended survival in people with many forms of cancer has become the rule rather than the exception. Multimodal treatments including surgery, radiation and chemotherapy place an intense burden on the patient and their family.

Previously, response to treatment was measured in terms of survival time and physician-rated treatment toxicity. More recently, QOL has emerged as the essence of broad-based assessment of the impact of disease and treatment. Many physicians initially attempt to measure QOL by measuring overt behaviour, because it is observable and measurable. These efforts fail because they neglect the underlying cognitive processes that mediate patient perception of QOL (Cella 1992). Individuals have a need to find meaning in their experience: 'man is not destroyed by suffering, but by suffering without meaning' (Frankl 1963).

QOL assessment is both subjective and multidimensional. Multidimensionality refers to the psychometric tradition of health status measurement; this includes, according to Cella (1992), physical, functional, emotional and social well-being. Cella emphasises that to date very little empirical work has been done to determine the relative importance of each of the major dimensions. QOL is said to have four major domains:

- functional well-being
- physical well-being
- emotional well-being
- social well-being.

Spirituality, while very important to some, has little importance to others; it also means different things to different people (Cella 1992).

WHY MEASURE QUALITY OF LIFE?

The perception exists that in the United States, and to a lesser extent in Canada, aggressive anti-cancer treatments are sometimes continued

In palliative care, symptom control rather than curative intervention is important. Measuring quality of life is one way of identifying the potential for enhancing a patient's QOL with new medical and non-medical interventions.

Recent improvements in the prevention and management of the side effects of chemotherapy and reduction in the length of hospital stay may make palliative chemotherapy more acceptable. New less-toxic chemotherapy regimens are being developed which may shift the argument in favour of chemotherapy. The use of QOL measurement during and following treatment is a way of accumulating evidence. Only a few studies have actually included the QOL measure in their assessment of palliative care (Bullinger 1992).

Bullinger (1992) goes on to say that it is necessary to have unobtrusive, clear-cut, standardised and well-tested instruments with which to investigate specific questions. This seems to suggest that QOL can be standardised. Bullinger identifies the importance of having an instrument which is reliable and valid and also sensitive to change. Validity suggests a test measures what it is intended to measure. We must not forget that the cultural and professional model used to define and conceptualise the topic may influence this.

The Karnofsky performance index (KPS) is the most frequently cited 'quality of life' measure found in medical literature (Fallowfield 1990). This scale was actually developed to determine the nursing requirements on a ward, not as a QOL measurement tool. It measures the patient's ability to self-care. Clark & Fallowfield (1986) point out the absurdities of the scale, which assumes if a person is not mobile they have a poor QOL. Using this scale, a breast cancer patient who is fully mobile may score 80%; emotional distress is not considered.

Bullinger (1992) also discusses reliability. A reliable test may not be a good test, since merely stating that a test measures something reliably tells us little unless we know what that something is: therefore, is the test valid?

It is unlikely that any one test will be suitable for all the different age groups and medical specialties. For example, some tests have a number of questions relating to sexual functioning, which may be inappropriate to some populations of patients, even offensive. There are a number of generic QOL measurement tools and a number which have been specifically developed for cancer research. Generic instruments often measure mood, function or symptoms: for example, the Rotterdam Symptom Check List (de Haes et al 1990); or the quality-adjusted time without symptoms or toxicity (Q-TWIST) analysis, developed by Gelber et al (1996). The disease-specific instruments usually measure physical, psychological and social dimensions of QOL. Measures that are disease-specific have been developed by the European Organisation for Research and Treatment of Cancer (EORTC) Quality of Life Unit.

The choice of instrument depends on the purpose of the QOL study. Three types of research questions can be distinguished according to Bullinger (1992):

- documentation of effects after treatment
- comparison of effects over time of different treatments
- evaluation of effects on individual patients.

QOL assessment can also be used to assess need. Christ & Siegel (1990) used telephone interviews to identify the need for ongoing pain relief, interpersonal contact and professional psychological support for cancer sufferers.

One might question the appropriateness of existing QOL measurement instruments for use in palliative care. One could argue that the philosophical and spiritual dimensions require greater consideration. In the final stages of life the frame of reference for measuring QOL may change rapidly. Morris et al (1992), in a study involving 300 cancer patients, identified deterioration in QOL, particularly during the last few weeks of life. However, 20% of the patients continued to rate their QOL as favourable, even during this time.

Instruments are available that attempt to measure the existential value of life for seriously ill people; for example, 'the meaning of life score' (Warner & Williams 1987).

The existential domain

In an interesting paper by Cohen & Mount (1992) using case study vignettes to illustrate QOL issues, the authors identify the diversity of factors moulding human perception of 'quality time'. They identify paradoxes in which the patients' perception of QOL is the opposite to that expected. For some patients, confrontation with death results in clarification of their understanding of human existence. This supports Frankl's (1963) thesis that a sense of QOL depends upon the perception of personal meaning. There may be an increase in perceived QOL in spite of coexisting suffering. The significance of meaning and transcendence as determinants of QOL has been recognised by Cassell (1991) as a way in which one may be restored to wholeness after injury to personhood. This recognition has resulted in the development of instruments that seek to assess a sense of purpose, meaning and spiritual aspects to life. While the goals of palliative care are acknowledged to include spiritual care, many investigators have chosen to ignore this aspect of human experience (Cohen & Mount 1992). Aaronson (1990) suggests that notions such as 'life satisfaction and happiness' have been judged to be distal to the goals of health care, and therefore seem inappropriate criteria against which to measure the efficacy of medical intervention. Schipper (1990) supports Aaronson in objecting to the inclusion of the existential and spiritual dimensions in QOL measurement tools. Mount & Scott (1983) point out that any QOL measure in palliative care must reflect meaning of life; by ignoring meaning and transcendence, we ignore a dimension central to palliative care.

The spiritual dimension of life may be described as having two planes: the horizontal and the vertical. The horizontal plane is about this life's concerns, such as finding satisfaction and meaning of life; this is often called the existential dimension. The vertical plane describes our relation with God or a higher being and may involve religion or religious practice (Palontzian & Ellison 1982). It can be seen that all patients have existential needs; the dying patient may have unmet needs on one or both planes. If we don't ask, we won't know.

Instruments which do include the spiritual dimension of life

1. MacMasters Health Index Questionnaire (Chambers et al 1992)
2. Quality of Life Index (Ferrans & Powers 1985)
3. The MacAdams and Smith Instrument (1987)
4. The Purpose of Life Test (Crumbaugh & Maholick 1964)
5. The Meaning of Life Score (Warner & Williams 1987)
6. The McGill Quality of Life Questionnaire (Cohen & Mount 1997).

> **Reflection point**
>
> How important do you feel it is to include the existential domain in QOL measurement?

ETHICAL CONSIDERATIONS

Ethical issues surrounding the inclusion of dying patients in research requires much consideration. While most care professionals are aware of the potential harm in clinical trials, many believe the so-called 'soft' research is relatively benign. The notion of informed consent requires consideration. The vulnerable dependent palliative care patient may feel unable to refuse to participate; they are unable to 'vote with their feet' if they change their minds. It is also not acceptable to treat vulnerable people as means to an end; most patients participating in palliative care research will not benefit from the research. Informed consent implies that patients are not being used as means to an end and are willing to participate. Many researchers claim that patients enjoy the extra attention they receive by being involved (Fallowfield et al 1986).

de Raeve (1994) questions this assumption, exploring the benefits and possible harm in implied informed consent. The researcher offers time, a listening ear, a nonjudgemental approach and interest; this can be a godsend to the lonely or anxious patient. The patient may perceive the researcher in the role of the therapist or counsellor and disclose intimate and sensitive information. If the researcher is also a nurse: to whom is the patient giving consent? the nurse or the researcher?

Additional questions need to be asked about such a relationship: how will this relationship be terminated and what support is given to the researcher? The type and nature of supervision given to researchers in this situation require some consideration.

Arunda (1995) cites Kellehear (1989), who offers a different argument. On a superficial level the notion of harm may include behaviour such as crying and distress. However, such behaviour is not uncommon in the dying and the bereaved; they are an inevitable part of grief and loss. The researcher would have difficulty in knowing if the distress was caused by the questions or the loss. Those who work with the dying know that not talking about painful subjects does not make the pain go away, or make it less painful. Crying and sharing an experience can be therapeutic. Aranda (1995) states that there may well be a therapeutic value in the research process which is frequently unreported. There is a need to extend our knowledge and understanding of the illness experience and issues around death and dying. It is important to improve the care of this vulnerable group of patients. This would be difficult to achieve without involving the palliative care patient. The opportunity for patients to voice their opinions and beliefs can demonstrate to those concerned that their views are valued, and that they can contribute to research which can help others. QOL research aims to improve care; it is unlikely to succeed without the help of the patients. Involving vulnerable groups in research should not be undertaken lightly. There is a need to explore and eliminate any potential harm, ensuring that such issues are discussed during the protocol development stage. Researchers undertaking such research should understand the palliative care philosophy and the principles of palliative care. The patient is always more important than the data collection and the research. The preparation, supervision and support of the researcher should also be given consideration.

THE CHALLENGE TO NURSING

The preservation of human dignity is or should be a central issue in everyday nursing. The relief of pain and suffering is one of the fundamental ways in which this is achieved. Pain and symptom relief is one of the primary aims of palliative care, and is a value shared with bioethics. But palliative care is more than pain and symptom management. The challenge to nursing, nurse education and nursing research is to develop the concept of QOL into a working model of care. QOL from the patient's perspective must become the goal of care. Dudgeon (1992) identifies the differences in the biomedical model and the illness model used by nurses, suggesting that nurses are concerned with the psychosocial aspects of disease and illness in addition to the physical symptoms. People who are sick experience their unwellness in a physical, psychological, social and spiritual way. According to Dudgeon the QOL conceptual model is intended to provide a broad biopsychosocial paradigm for making evaluations from the patient's perspective.

When cure is no longer an option, caring becomes the primary objective. Caring is a concept that is fundamental in nursing. Grealish (1997) suggests that in some situations the operationalisation of this concept is difficult. One reason offered by Grealish (1997) is the narrow view of nursing practice offered by the dominant biomedical model. The ethical nature of nursing should be grounded in an ethic which is broader than that of bioethics. A QOL approach to assessment, care planning and evaluation would be further strengthened if nurses adopted an ethic of care. Grealish (1997) argues that palliative care nurses are well placed to develop a lead in the field of nursing ethics.

The ethic of care provides a framework for understanding the ethical nature of the nurse–patient relationship in a way which reflects the patients' view of their QOL. This could further strengthen a QOL approach. The ethic of care is based on the following assumptions about what are desirable goals of care:

1. the alleviation of suffering
2. the preservation of human dignity
3. fidelity, or promise-keeping
4. patient as expert
5. interdependence.

The alleviation of suffering is consistent with the primary aim of palliative care. It must be remembered that suffering is a much broader concept than pain and has various dimensions (see Salt 1997). The preservation of dignity is central to palliative care; fidelity or promise-keeping is also essential in the nurse–patient relationship as breaking a promise abuses trust; both concepts deserve further exploration beyond the scope of this essay. Using the ethic of care approach places the patient in the position of an expert; this view is grounded in the value of human dignity. Patients' views are valued and sought; they know more about how they experience their disease than the professional does. We no longer label patients as being compliant or non-compliant; they are choosing a way of being that reflects their personal beliefs and values. Case study 16.1 may illustrate how important it is to seek the patient's view.

Interdependence assumes that the patient is a competent adult. For patients who are terminally ill and dependent, this autonomy is threatened. Frequently, health professionals communicate with each other and the patient's family, neglecting the patient's view. This causes conflict in the patient–nurse relationship. Using an ethic of care approach demands that all meaning is co-constructed between patient and nurse. This involves listening, negotiating and mutual disclosure. According to Grealish (1997), consultation with the family members is then more straightforward, because the patient's views have been explored and clearly developed. It is possible that the use of QOL assessment could provide a framework in which the patient's views could be identified.

Working in this way, the nurse seeks to reconceptualise and describe the patient's symptoms in a way that has meaning for the patient and their family.

Such an approach was used by Ferrell et al (1992) in a study to identify the QOL issues for bone marrow transplant survivors (BMTS). The

CASE STUDY 16.1

SEEKING THE PATIENT'S VIEW

When interviewing hospice patients to establish how well they felt their pain was being managed I noticed an elderly man walking continuously up and down the corridor with his Zimmer frame. Discussion with Harold revealed that he was an 82-year-old man with prostate cancer who had come to the hospice for pain control 2 weeks earlier and was due to be discharged home the following day. 'They only care about your cancer pain in here', he told me. It transpired that Harold had an in-growing toe nail which was painful when he walked. Harold had informed the staff two or three times since admission about his toe nail. He told me: 'I'm not afraid to die, but I want to die at home'. Harold believed that it was essential that he stay 'on his feet' and be independent as he had lived alone since his wife died 10 years ago. His cancer pain was well managed but his toe nail was a source of pain and concern. Walking, he said, was 'hellish'. I suggested he exercise less as it was so painful (7 on a visual analogue scale when walking). Walking was so important to Harold that he felt he must maintain his activity level. This example illustrates the importance of understanding what the priorities of the patient are. Harold was not worried about his cancer or dying; his mobility was his main concern. An in-growing toe nail may seem trivial to us but it was a major concern to him and threatened his quality of life.

patients were asked six open-ended questions. Analysis of the data resulted in a conceptual model which can be used to describe and distinguish the various dimensions of the illness experience of BMTS, providing a more holistic view than might have previously been available. A holistic approach to QOL assessment and measurement may provide the framework and focus of care which is patient-centred and based on the patient's perception and experience of illness. The use of the ethic of care model may strengthen this approach, as it supports the notion of patient as a competent adult and as an expert.

CONCLUSION

Quality of life is a complex changing multidimensional construct of various dimensions which may change in order of priority over time. QOL measurement can be used to evaluate medical and psychosocial interventions; it can also give insight into the patient's priorities and concerns. The sensitive use of QOL assessment may have therapeutic benefits: this merits further exploration. It is possible that the QOL interview could facilitate a meaningful discussion between the patient and nurse, in which the existential needs of the patient might be explored. The inclusion of dying patients in research requires careful consideration, in order to avoid exposing this vulnerable group to harm. However, the use

of QOL assessment as part of an ongoing evaluation of care may be justified in that it may improve the quality of care for the individual concerned, and improve the care of future patients.

With the patient's consent, such information may be subject to secondary analysis and used retrospectively in research without further burden to the patient. Many writers claim that the dying may find meaning in their suffering if they believe that they can somehow help others in the future: contributing to QOL research may be one way of doing this.

REFERENCES

Aaronson N K 1990 Quality of life research in cancer clinical trials. A need for common rules and language. Oncology 4(5): 59–66

Aranda S 1995 Conducting research with the dying: ethical considerations and experience. International Journal of Palliative Nursing 1(1): 41–47

Axelsson B, Sjoden P 1998 Quality of life of cancer patients and their spouses in palliative home care. Palliative Medicine 12: 29–39

Berado D 1992 Quality of life across age and family stages. Journal of Palliative Care 8(3): 52–55

Biegel D E, Sales S, Schulz R 1991 Family caregiving in chronic illness. Newbury Park, California

Bowling A 1995 What things are important in people's lives. A survey of the public's judgements to inform scales of health related quality of life. Social Science and Medicine 41: 1447–1462

Bremnes R M, Anderson K, Wist E A 1995 Cancer patients' doctors and nurses vary in their willingness to undertake cancer chemotherapy. European Journal of Cancer 31A: 1955–1959

Brock D W (ed.) 1993 Quality of life measures in healthcare and medical ethics. In: Life and death. Cambridge University Press, Cambridge, pp. 268–324

Bullinger M 1992 Quality of life assessment in palliative care. Journal of Palliative Care 8(3): 34–39

Calman K C 1984 Quality of life in cancer patients. An hypothesis. Journal of Medical Ethics 10: 124–127

Cassell E J 1991 The nature of suffering and the goals of medicine. Oxford University Press, New York, pp. 37–43

Cella D 1992 Health, quality of life, the concept. Journal of Palliative Care 8(3): 8–13

Cella D F, Cherin E A 1988 Quality of life during and after cancer treatment. Comprehensive Therapy 14(5): 69–75

Chambers L W, MacDonald L A, Tugwell P, Buchanan W M, Krag 1992 Nursing diagnosis: an ethical analysis. MacMasters Health Index Questionnaire. Journal of Nursing Scholarship 22(2): 99–103

Christ G, Siegel K 1990 Monitoring quality of life needs in cancer patients. Cancer 65: 760–765

Clark A W, Fallowfield L J 1986 Quality of life measurements in patients with malignant disease: a review. Journal of the Royal Society of Medicine 79: 165–169

Coates A 1992 Application of quality of life measures in health care delivery. Journal of Palliative Care 8(3): 18–21

Cohen S R, Mount B 1992 Quality of life in terminal illness. Defining and measuring subjective well-being in the dying. Journal of Palliative Care 8(3): 40–45

Cohen S R, Mount B 1997 Validity of the McGill quality of life questionnaire in the palliative care setting. A multi-centred Canadian study demonstrating the importance of the existential domain. Palliative Medicine 6: 18–20

Crumbaugh J C, Maholick L T 1964 An experimental study in existentialism. The psychometric approach to Frankl's concept of nogenic neurosis. Journal of Clinical Psychology 20: 200–207

de Haes J C J, Knippenberg F C E, Neijit P 1990 Measuring psychological and physical distress in cancer patients: structure and application of the Rotterdam symptom checklist. British Journal of Cancer 62: 10348

de Raeve L 1994 Ethical issues in palliative care research. Palliative Medicine 8: 298–305

Douglas C 1992 For all the saints. British Medical Journal 304: 579

Dudgeon D 1992 Quality of life: a bridge between the biomedical model and illness models of medicine and nursing. Journal of Palliative Care 8(3): 14–17

Fallowfield L 1990 The quality of life the forgotten measurement. Human Horizon Series. Souvenir Press, London

Fallowfield L J, Baum M, Maguire G 1986 Do psychological studies upset patients? Journal of the Royal Society of Medicine 80: 59

Farquahar M 1995 Elderly people's definitions of quality of life. Social Science and Medicine 41: 1439–1446

Feil L, Hahn Winslow E H 1985 Moving to a nursing model. American Journal of Nursing October: 1100–1101

Ferrans C E, Powers M J 1985 Quality of life index. Development of psychometric properties. Advanced Nursing Science 8: 15–24

Ferrell B, Schmidt D, Rhiner M, Whitehead C, Fonbeun P, Forman S 1992 The meaning of quality of life for bone marrow transplant survivors. Cancer Nursing 15(3): 153–160

Frankl V E 1963 Man's search for meaning. New York Pocket Books, New York

Ganz P A, Lee J J, Sian J 1991 Quality of life assessment: an independent prognosis. Variable for Survival in Lung Cancer 67: 3131–3135

Gelber R D, Godhurst A, Coe B, Wieand H S, Schroeder G, Krook J 1996 A quality adjusted time without symptoms or toxicity (Q TWIST) analysis of adjuvant radiation and chemotherapy for resectable rectal cancer. Journal of National Cancer Institute 88: 1039–1045

Gill T M, Feinstein A R 1994 A critical appraisal of the quality of life measurement. Journal of the American Medical Association 272: 619–626

Grealish L 1997 Beyond Hippocrates: ethics in palliative care. International Journal of Palliative Nursing 3(3): 151–155

Hadorn D C 1991 The Oregon priority – setting exercise quality of life and public policy. Hastings Centre Report May/June: 11–16

Higginson I 1995 Outcome measures in palliative care. Working Party in Clinical Guidelines in Palliative Care. National Hospice Council, London

Hinton J 1994 Can home care maintain an acceptable quality of life for patients with terminal cancer and their relatives? Palliative Medicine 8: 183–196

Kellehear A 1989 Ethics and social research. In: Perry J (ed.) Doing field work, eight personal accounts of social research. Deakin University Press, Australia

MacAdam D B, Smith M 1987 An initial assessment of suffering in terminal illness. Palliative Medicine 1: 37–47

MacDonald N 1992 Quality of life in clinical and research palliative medicine. Journal of Palliative Care 8(3): 46–51

Mast M E 1995 Definition and measurement of quality of life in oncology. Nursing research: review and theoretical implications. Oncology Nursing Forum 22(6): 957–964

Mishel M H 1990 Reconceptualisation of the uncertainty in illness theory. Image: Journal of Nursing Scholarship 22: 254–256

Montazeri A, Gillis C R, McEwan J 1996 Measuring quality of life in oncology: Is it worthwhile? Experiences from the treatment of cancer. European Journal of Cancer Care 5: 168–175

Morris J, Cull A, Fallowfield L et al 1992 British Psychological Oncology Group Seventh Annual Conference. British Journal of Cancer 65: 136

Mount B M, Scott J F 1983 Whither hospice evaluation. Journal of Chronic Disease 36: 731–736

Padilla G V, Mishel M H, Grant M M 1992 Uncertainty, appraisal and quality of life. Quality of Life Research 1: 155–165

Palontzian R F, Ellison C W 1982 Loneliness, spiritual well-being and quality of life research and therapy. In: Peplau L A, Perriman D (eds) Loneliness: a source book of current theories. Wiley, New York

Parker G 1990 Spouse carers; Who's quality of life. In: Baldwin S, Godfrey C, Propper C (eds) Quality of life: perspectives and policies. Routledge, London, pp. 120–130

Salt S 1997 Towards a definition of suffering. European Journal of Palliative Care 4(2): 58–60

Schipper H 1990 Guidelines and caveats for quality of life: measurement in clinical practice and research. Oncology 4(5): 51–57

Schipper H 1992 Quality of life the final common pathway. Journal of Palliative Care 8(3): 5–7

Selai M L, Rosser R M 1993 Good quality, some methodological issues. Journal of the Royal Society of Medicine 86: 440–444

Selvin M L, Plant H, Lynch D, Drinkwater J, Gregory W M 1988 Who should measure quality of life, the doctor or the patient? British Journal of Cancer 57: 109–112

Tierney A L, Sladden S, Anderson J, King M, Llewellyn S 1994 Measuring the cost and quality of palliative care: a discussion paper. Palliative Medicine 8: 273–281

Warner S C, Williams J I 1987 The meaning of life scale: determining the reliability and validity of measure. Journal of Chronic Disease 40(6): 503–512

Weeks J 1992 Quality of life assessment: performance status upstaged? Journal of Clinical Oncology 10: 1827–1829

17

Looking after yourself

Fiona Setch

INTRODUCTION

I say, I say, I say
How do you stop a conversation at a party?
I don't know, how do you stop a conversation at a party?
By admitting that you work with people who are dying . . .

(Fiona Setch:
On numerous occasions from 1989–today)

Does that strike a popular chord for you?

Death, dying, bereavement and loss remain taboo subjects for most of Western society and, within health care, the traditional medical model still views death as a failure to cure. Vachon (1997) highlights that stress and burn out exist in palliative care but are generally less than in other specialties. This may be due to the recognition of the inherent stress of working within palliative care which resulted in support programmes being built into the work at the beginning.

But things have changed somewhat since 'the beginning', as specialist palliative care units are responding and changing to meet the needs of not only those patients with cancer, AIDS and motor neurone disease (MND) but also with other illnesses such as end-stage cardiac, renal and neurological diseases. There are increasing numbers of younger patients with complex family dynamics being referred to palliative care services.

The aim of this chapter is to provide you with the opportunity to identify the specific stressors within palliative care and how they impact on your work.

To explore your existing support strategies and how these may be further developed to enhance your work, we include professional support mechanisms such as training, clinical supervision and reflective practice as well as your own individual personal support needs. There will be the opportunity to review your own practice and to perform your own personal action plan at the end of the chapter.

Reading this chapter will provide you with the time and space to think about your own support needs. There are several exercises that you can complete to explore the issues involved in looking after yourself. To do this you will find the following useful:

- paper
- different coloured highlighter pens
- time
- space
- to be open and honest with yourself
- a friend/colleague to discuss issues that may come up for you
- a sense of humour!

Paper and coloured pens are used as life is seldom black and white; you may want to highlight parts of your experiences.

There is an important principle that I would encourage you to think about while working your way through this chapter: there is no such thing as better than or less than – just different. That is, there are different ways of working, coping, involving, caring and your way is quite unique to you; it is quite simply *your way*.

In the film 'Dead Poets Society', Robin Williams portrays a teacher who challenges conventional teaching methods. During one scene he asks his students to stand on their desks rather than sit at them, to view the classroom from another angle. During this chapter, I would like to invite you to look at your ideas of support from a different perspective. Whatever your role is within palliative care nursing, the aim of this chapter is that you will have an increased awareness of what your own individual support needs are.

Stotter (1992) suggests that the quality of care given to patients can rely on the extent to which carers feel cared for. Staff support should be an integral part of specialist palliative care.

This chapter, 'Looking after yourself', is one that focuses on empowerment and personal responsibility, as only you know what you need to support you in your role. As nurses, it is our individual right to enable us to bring comfort and hope!

WHAT IS STRESS?

Stress can best be explained by the illustration shown in Figure 17.1. I am sure you will be adding a few more labels to the list.

McKenzie (1994, p. 3) defines stress as:

High demands plus high constraints, plus low support = stress

During 1997, the Government commissioned a report about the well-being of health care workers called: 'Improving the Health of the NHS Workforce' (Williams 1998). This report revealed new information about the ill health of both the environment and those providing care in the NHS, and amongst its recommendations was that staff should be encouraged to look after their own health. Caregivers need to recognise that it takes a whole person to respond day after day to the holistic needs of other people. Within health care, work overload, lack of resources and staff shortages have become major stressors in general health care, but what are the specific stressors in palliative care?

STRESS SPECIFIC TO PALLIATIVE CARE

Outside pressures are known as stressors. They contribute to the physiological stress reaction that involves complex metabolic, endocrine, cardiovascular and neurological adaptations of the body to stress-inducing events, which can eventually lead to illness or exhaustion. Problems arise when stress is maintained over a lengthy period of time, which can result in burn out. Battle fatigue and burn out are terms specifically used to describe staff stress when caring for patients who are dying.

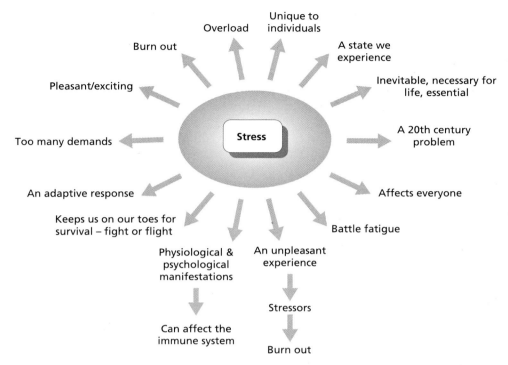

Figure 17.1 What is stress?

Language is extremely powerful. How often do we read media headlines such as:

Linda McCartney loses valiant fight against cancer?

There is an implicit assumption of failure in this headline, which can act as a stressor in caring for dying people. For patients, words like cancer and death are tainted with so many images of horror (Fig. 17.2). Few people in society actually know what happens when someone dies.

Part of the 'battle fatigue' described by Vachon (1997) is the constantly normalising and processing of the patient and their loved ones' anxieties – as well as our own feelings as human beings, who happen to work as nurses.

Murray Parkes (1998) advocates that in order to help those who are dying, we must be prepared to get close to them, to share their fears and to stay with them in their fear. This involves a deep level of communication which offers the double-edged sword of being both an absolute privilege and a sometimes painful experience.

Twycross (1995) suggests that there are several challenges that are inevitable in palliative care:

- facing your own mortality
- facing your own limitations personally and professionally
- sharing control
- learning to be with patients rather than doing things for them
- dealing honestly with your emotions.

(Adapted from Twycross 1995)

Some of these issues are illustrated in Case studies 17.1 and 17.2.

Personal reflections of the case studies

In the two case studies, I was carer, friend and a large part of Sue's support system while at work being charge nurse, clinical supervisor and part of several staff members' support systems. In relation to the patient Colin I was nurse, carer and confidant and support giver to his family and partner.

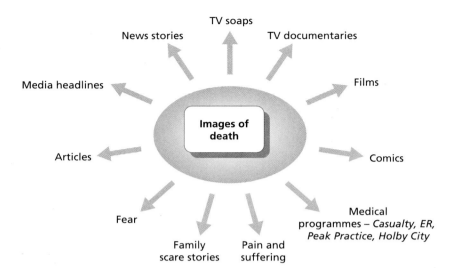

Figure 17.2 Images of death.

I am sharing my personal experience as I learned an invaluable lesson about the absolute importance of personal support, support systems and the essential role of clinical supervision. Although, in retrospect, it wasn't until some time had passed that I became aware of what my own needs were. I am well aware that I came very close to burn out and was in danger of becoming:

- physically and emotionally exhausted
- feeling worn out
- losing my enthusiasm
- doubting my abilities to provide leadership
- doubting my abilities to care for patients
- cynical, disillusioned and angry
- dreading going to work.

The turning point for me was my clinical supervision session, during which I became empowered to identify what I needed to do to avoid becoming further stressed. Clinical supervision was then and is today, in my current role, one of my main support mechanisms and I will be discussing clinical supervision in more detail later in this chapter.

STAFF SUPPORT

'What does staff support mean to you?' was a question I was asked to think about during a workshop at a conference on staff support in palliative care.

Assisting people to achieve, there never seems to be enough, priority, facilitate, listening, fascination and perplexity . . . were amongst the responses, but the one that captured my imagination was:

Not that old dinosaur again!

Interesting, I thought, and was immediately transported to the film 'Jurassic Park'; thinking what type of dinosaur would I choose to resemble my idea of staff support:

- Perhaps a diplodoccus or a tyrannosaurus rex?
- What would your dinosaur look like?

Each of us has our own individual experience of life, our nursing, our own values and expectations – therefore, our 'dinosaurs' will vary in some unique way. The notion of staff support being 'that old dinosaur again' may be about the concept of support having been around for a long, long time.

CASE STUDY 17.1

CARING FOR SUE

Sue is a 33-year-old nurse. She had been diagnosed with non-Hodgkin's lymphoma 3 years ago while working and travelling in New Zealand, following which she worked in Somalia for Save the Children Fund for 2 years. Sue returned to the UK, was in the process of buying her home in Bristol and was 2 months into her Health Visiting Diploma when the lymphoma became aggressive.

Following chemotherapy and a period or remission of 3 months, the lymphoma re-occurred in the form of a cerebral lymphoma.

Sue underwent 3 months of intensive radiotherapy and chemotherapy; as a result of these treatments she had numerous admissions to the same oncology ward, where she got to know the staff very well.

Sue's immediate carers were her partner of 5 years, Richard, who had been working as a doctor overseas, and two close friends who were nurses. All three carers were particularly involved in Sue's care.

Sue was in denial about her health, having fertility treatment and planning a beach holiday in Greece in 3 months' time with Richard. She deteriorated suddenly, lapsed into unconsciousness and died 24 hours later in the arms of her partner – her two friends camped out in the day room. All three carers were very stoical and appeared to be 'holding it together'.

Sue's friends requested that they care for her after death. They washed and dressed her in her favourite clothes and put her make-up and jewellery on. All unnecessary clinical equipment was cleared away from Sue's room and replaced by aromatherapy oils and music. . . . When Sue's room was ready, they invited the nursing staff to say goodbye. After they had completed this, the carers spent their own private time with Sue and left the hospital ward.

1. If you were one of the nurses on this oncology unit, involved in caring for Sue, what would some of the issues of care be for you?
2. What feelings do you think you would be experiencing during Sue's care?

Issues	*Feelings*
Sue: a young, inspirational woman	Sadness
Age identification	This could be me/one of my friends
Peer – a fellow nurse	Personal identification
Personal identification	Help!
Sue starting a new life-career, new home	This is so unjust!
Partner – a doctor – knowledgeable	Challenged, Sue and carers knowledgeable
Close friends are nurses	How to help carers
Carers very stoical	How would I cope?
Sue's denial of illness, death	Does she need to know her reality?
Fertility treatment	Can only be there for Sue to talk
Length of hospital visits	Privilege to know Sue – but hard
Five months of intensive nursing	Going to be really hard when Sue dies
Sue very friendly with staff	Sharing of intensive time with Sue
Sudden deterioration	Quick death, better quality of life, relief
Carers took control at time of death	Sadness for self, Richard and friends Slightly disempowered
Carers performed last offices	On reflection best thing for them Privileged to be able to facilitate this
Carers invited nurses to say goodbye	What a beautiful death! Sadness

Whose responsibility is it to provide support? Individual vs. organisational

Individual and organisational support is illustrated in Figure 17.3.

Vachon (1997) suggests that dealing with job stress is not solely the responsibility of either the individual or the organisation. Effective coping strategies require the use of personal and environmental coping mechanisms. Caregivers are twice as likely to report to personal coping strategies as being helpful in dealing with occupational stress than organisational strategies.

The organisation that you work for may well provide you with many things – employment, salary, colleagues, working environment, educational opportunities and occupational health – but unless you are aware of your own support needs, you may not feel supported. Individual nurses who expect their organisations to be their main support are setting themselves and their organisation up to fail. So how do you identify what your support needs are?

CASE STUDY 17.2

CARE FOR THE CARER

Fiona, a 28-year-old staff nurse, receives a letter from one of her best friends, Sue, who is currently nursing in New Zealand. The letter contained the news that she has been diagnosed with non-Hodgkin's lymphoma but not to worry, as it is not aggressive and she is asymptomatic.

During the next 3 years, they correspond regularly and meet up whenever Sue is home. Fiona is now working as a nurse in a London residential unit, caring for people with HIV/AIDS.

Sue talks to Fiona about living with cancer, sharing her disease progress and her hopes and fears. Their close friendship deepens.

Two years later, Fiona is promoted to charge nurse on the unit. She enjoys her work tremendously, finding it extremely challenging, managing a 24-bed unit, being part of a dynamic charge nurse team, being a clinical supervisor of a team of 10 trained nurses as well as some patient care. Sue has recently returned to the UK and is starting her health visiting training in Bristol.

Sue's cancer suddenly becomes aggressive. Several months later, Sue's condition deteriorates suddenly. She is very depressed and Fiona spends as much time with Sue as she can. As a result, Fiona is physically tired and emotionally drained. Fiona recently spent a week's holiday visiting Sue and accompanying her for radiotherapy treatments, as well as 'girlie things' like watching Wimbledon tennis together, shopping, eating out and many hours of talking and just spending time together.

On her first shift back at work after visiting Sue, Colin, a patient whom Fiona had known and nursed for 4 years, was admitted for terminal care. Fiona had been his 'key nurse' in her previous job.

Following hand over, Fiona receives a telephone call from her mother with the unexpected news that an old family friend has died suddenly. Fiona has a clinical supervision appointment with her line manager at 3pm.

1. What are the issues facing Fiona?
2. How do you think that clinical supervision could be supportive to Fiona?

1.   Issues facing Fiona

- Sadness at the illness of Sue.
- Sue's illness has brought their existing friendship even closer.
- Personal identification.
- Emotionally tired due to job stress and supporting Sue.
- Over-extending personal resources, spending a week's holiday with ill friend.
- Overwhelming situation – on return to work.
- Sadness at Colin's deterioration in health.
- Feeling unable to cope with the sudden death of an old family friend.
- Feeling guilty that she wasn't coping.
- Wanting to be there for Colin and his family – but knowing she would burst into tears . . .
- Feeling guilty.
- Feelings of inadequacy.

2.   How could clinical supervision support Fiona?

- Providing a confidential space, uninterrupted, away from the unit, to focus on what was occurring.
- Space to focus on the impact of how personal life was affecting professional practice.
- Reflection, critical incident of Colin's deterioration and how despite being involved in Colin's care for so long, another team member could be his key nurse.
- Direction to 'practice what she preached' to the staff that she supervised and to take some time out to attend family friend's funeral and to be able to be there when Sue died.
- The opportunity to explore and review her support systems and an action plan how she was going to cope with the challenging time ahead.
- Validation of Fiona as a human being and her skills as a professional nurse.
- Acknowledgement that this was a very difficult, painful time – and that, that was the way it was – but it would pass.

Recognising your dinosaur – what are your personal support needs?

During times of stress, our network of support can help us to cope with the demands placed upon us. Our contacts can act as a buffer, by relieving us of some of the pressure – or as a safety valve, by providing an outlet for feelings.

Support network mind map

No man is an island, entire of itself,
Every man is a piece of the continent, a part of the main.
(John Donne 1571–1631)

For this exercise you will need:
   A large piece of paper, pens.

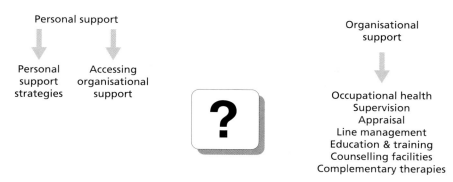

Figure 17.3   Individual and organisational support.

Step 1

Write your name in the middle of the page and draw a circle around it.

Step 2

Think of your existing support structures.

Draw in the main branches – these are the main categories that make up your network; label them. For example, see Figure 17.4.

Step 3

Having identified the main categories, the next step involves drawing smaller branches from the large ones, with specific people who give you support (Fig. 17.5). Your named people can be anyone who supports you. For example:

- *Work*: Your manager, team members, other colleagues, peers, a support group, the organisation.
- *Family and friends*: Your partner, parents, children, siblings, pets, extended family, friends.
- *Professional*: Union, GP, supervisor, counsellor, aromatherapist.
- *Interest*: Social, church, sports, education, charity work, club.

Only include the names of people that you would actively seek support from.

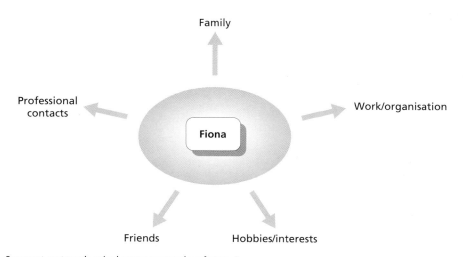

Figure 17.4   Support network mind map: example of step 2.

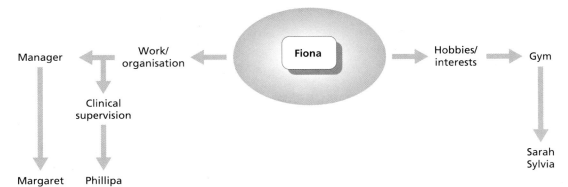

Figure 17.5   Support network mind map: example of step 3.

Step 4

With different coloured pens, write a 'W' next to the names of people who help you to resolve your work-related problems.

Step 5

Reflect on your support network. For someone to be able to support you, they need to know what your needs are. For example, sometimes you may need to simply tell the story of an event, without interruptions, questions or suggestions. Whereas, on another occasion, you will need/ want to be challenged.

On both occasions, the person listening is not telepathic; therefore, you need to communicate your needs clearly, otherwise you could unknow-ingly be setting both yourself and the person lis-tening to fail and end up feeling frustrated, angry and even less supported than you felt originally.

In order to assert your needs, you need to be clear about who is capable of providing what to you in specific examples. Complete Table 17.1 to identify who is involved in your support struc-ture.

Having completed this exercise:

- What are your initial thoughts on your individual support system?
- Does your support system give you the right type of support, with a balance between work and emotional issues?
- Are there enough people in it?

- What gaps exist if any?
- Are you in danger of making too many demands on too few people?
- Are there any surprises?
- What changes would you like to make?
- How will you go about it?

Table 17.1   Support structure

Types of support	Person who provides support
Accepting Someone who listens to you, nonjudgmentally and without giving advice	
Personal support Unconditional support for you even though they may not be in agreement with what you are doing. Your own personal backing group!	
Personal challenge Someone who asks you incisive questions, checking out your attitudes, feelings and behaviour	
Work-oriented support and challenge Someone who knows your job, can help you identify strengths and cope with difficulties	
Crisis work A skilled professional who can listen appropriately: e.g. counsellor, occupational health nurse	

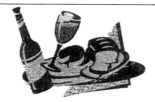

The Support Menu

Starter

Peer Support

Reflective Diary

Quiet Space . . . Time for Yourself

Exercise

Planning a Holiday

Main Course

Reflection in Action

Reflective Practice

Clinical Supervision

Annual Appraisal

Education & Training

Critical Incident Reflection

Coaching

Counselling

Sweet

Support Group

Teaching

Aromatherapy

Social Outing – a Drink, Meal or Coffee

'One of your Treats'

Being on Holiday

SUPPORT MENU

Earlier in the chapter, I mentioned the film 'Dead Poets Society'. Like Robin Williams' teacher, I would like to invite you to stand on your desk and view your support from a different perspective.

You have just identified your existing support strategies – this is an excellent starting point to think about looking after yourself – as if you are not well supported yourself, how can you support others effectively?

A method of thinking about your support strategies is to envisage options like an enticing restaurant menu. Imagine you are visiting your favourite restaurant. You open the menu and are faced with a sumptuous choice of starters, main courses and sweets. On some occasions you may want to choose a starter and main course or on others just a main course or go for the full works – starter, main course and sweet! I would like to present to you the Support Menu.

Examples from the starter menu might be writing in your reflective diary, or it may involve a quiet 5 minutes' relaxation. From the main course menu, education and training can be tremendously supportive. It is my observation that issues-based multidisciplinary training provides an excellent forum for constructive, supportive teamwork, as the comments taken from a 1-day experiential 'Caring for the Dying Course' illustrate.

What have been the benefits of attending this session?

- Sharing experiences with others.
- An increased awareness of my own feelings, surrounding death and dying.
- Time to focus on the activities of daily working life that have become normal.
- Time out to discuss the stresses of caring for the dying.
- Time out together to think and explore.
- A space for personal reflection.
- Knowing that most of my feelings are shared by others.
- Time out from the working environment and sharing a good laugh with colleagues.

Are there any changes you intend to make to your practice as a result of attending this training?

- To support each other more – demonstrate that we are there for each other.
- Allow more time to think quietly and gather thoughts.
- Attend reflective practice more often.
- Try to accept and give a higher priority to my own needs.
- Arranging agreed time to support colleagues and not just snatching a minute or so.
- Not to rely on bumping into a supportive colleague in the corridor for support anymore – making time for each other.

From my own Support Menu I would like to share a starter, main course and sweet. As a starter I suggest the pocket-sized self-help books: *Take Care of Yourself* (Sach 1997) and *The Little Book of Calm* (Wilson 1996). I find these texts both inspirational and very practical, as they are filled with exercises and 'thoughts for the day'.

Rest your fingers

One of my favourite exercises that I practise myself and with others is 'rest your fingers'. Ensure that you are sitting comfortably, both feet on the floor and take a deep breath in and slowly exhale. Close your eyes. Gently rest your thumbs and fingers of one hand against the thumbs and fingertips of the other, with just the lightest touch. Breathe slowly and count to 60 and invite the calm to be with you! (Adapted from *The Little Book of Calm* – Wilson 1996.)

My main course choices are reflection in action and clinical supervision.

Reflection in action

This is a tool that can be used in preparation for clinical supervision, as part of reflective practice or as a stand-alone critical incident review. Think of a critical incident and complete the following format (Table 17.2); it will help you clarify your position and evaluate what the learning was in it for you.

Table 17.2 Reflection in action (Sweetenham 1997)

R	**Recognise significant thoughts/feelings** What are you thinking? How are you feeling?
E	**Explore the significant elements** What is significant in your thoughts/ feelings? About the context of the situation?
F	**Focus on your response** How did you respond to the situation? How do you feel about your response?
L	**List the relevant underlying knowledge/experience/assumptions** What prior knowledge/experience/ assumptions lead you to respond in this way?
E	**Evaluate the validity of that knowledge/experience/assumptions** Did that prior knowledge/experience/ assumptions help you?
C	**Clarify what you have learned** What does this new learning do to your previous knowledge/experience/ assumptions?
T	**Transfer this learning to new situations** What will the new learning help you do in the future?

Clinical supervision

What do you know about clinical supervision? Take a few moments to answer this short quiz:

1. What is clinical supervision?
2. What are the functions of clinical supervision?
3. What are the benefits of clinical supervision?
4. What might be the blocks to clinical supervision?
5. What are some of the issues or challenges specific to working in palliative care that you think clinical supervision could help with?

1. What is clinical supervision?

There are numerous definitions of clinical supervision which include the following key themes:

- a process
- a regular, protected time
- a confidential space
- a facilitated reflection on clinical practice
- it enables the supervisee to achieve, sustain and develop high-quality practice
- a supervisee-led agenda
- a part of lifelong learning.

Bond & Holland (1998) conclude that clinical supervision should continue throughout a nurse's career, in whatever direction: clinical practice, research, education or management.

2. What are the functions of clinical supervision?

Your list may include:

- self-awareness
- personal management
- problem solving
- support
- education
- reflection
- analysis of situations
- planning
- development.

3. What are the benefits of clinical supervision?

- a 'sounding out space', confidentiality
- experience of a supportive, confidential relationship
- improve patient care by reflecting on practice, looking at skills, achievements and challenging situations, focusing on self
- provides clarity of direction: sets aims and objectives
- the opportunity to take 'time out', take a step back to reflect
- valuing personal achievements.

4. What might be the blocks to clinical supervision?

- lack of knowledge
- lack of trust and confidentiality
- time
- fear that 'it' will be challenging
- new concept
- more change
- lack of enthusiasm
- it may 'open up a can of worms'
- being judged
- who will do it?

Fears and concerns are normal with any new change or process. It is important to acknowledge fears and concerns, while exploring them thoroughly.

5. Specific issues and challenges of working in palliative care that clinical supervision can help with

- the curse of perfectionism – are you ever too hard on yourself?
- younger patients with complex social and psychological problems
- personal identification with patients
- multiple complex problems
- euthanasia
- many skilled staff may be involved in one patient – problems of power, feeling deskilled, communication problems
- intense time in patients' lives – that you work with day in and day out
- multiple bereavements
- working with death, dying, bereavement and loss – day in day out
- impact on personal life
- when problems in personal life – how do these impact on professional life? As evident in the two case studies
- being involved in a person's dying – privilege and pain.

Within palliative care, whatever our roles, we all strive for the very best for our patients. Perhaps it is because we are focusing on quality of life with a short time span? Are we caretakers of a living museum? Trying to ensure that the whole scene – patient, family and carers – have the best of everything, and our patients are remembered exactly as they want to be?

From my personal experiences of being both clinical supervisee and clinical supervisor, I believe that clinical supervision is an essential component of nursing. If you are not receiving clinical supervision, ask yourself the question why not? I suggest you find out what is available in your area of work.

All it takes is for two people to start talking about clinical supervision; obviously, you need to know about the concept and principles and there are some excellent resources available. A good way to begin is to find someone who has experience of clinical supervision or is interested in the concept – if you wait for others to provide it, you may be waiting a long time; so *carpe diem* – seize the day!

From my sweet menu I would like to share with you *10 treats*. Close your eyes and think of 10 things that you like doing for yourself that do not involve a lot of either time or money. Write down your list, which may include:

- a relaxing bath
- gardening
- walking the dog
- stroking your cat
- listening to a relaxation tape
- fishing
- watching a favourite TV programme
- cooking
- listening to music.

When you have compiled your list, look at it and visualise yourself enjoying your individual daily treats. Imagine how very happy and relaxed you feel when you do them.

Try and do at least one every day and enjoy treating yourself.

This exercise was the gift of Jim Kukendyall, a clinical psychologist who facilitated a ward-based support group that I was a member of.

SO WHAT NEXT?

During this chapter, I have outlined specific stressors within palliative care nursing. I chose to share my own personal experiences, as I believe in leading by example. By sharing my experience of how specific issues and challenges of working in palliative care affected me, I hope that it may help you in your work.

You also have had the opportunity to explore your existing support strategies and I have provided some examples of alternative strategies that you may choose to think about.

PERSONAL ACTION PLANNING

During the process of reflection, after having an experience and concluding from it, it is important to learn from this experience and plan for the next time.

There will be some very practical steps that you can take immediately, such as:

- identifying your existing support strategies
- giving yourself permission to think about yourself before thinking of supporting others.

There will be other steps that may take some time such as finding a clinical supervisor and starting clinical supervision.

A useful way of formalising these thoughts is to write them down as a personal action plan (Fig. 17.6).

These approaches may not seem appropriate for you and you may need to take some risks. My challenge to you is to take the time for yourself, reflect on the process, and I can guarantee it will improve your quality of work life, which has a knock-on effect on your whole life.

I would like to share a poem that has given me much inspiration since I heard it at a nursing conference in 1991.

Personal Action Plan

My current situation

I feel I am unsupported

What I would like it to be

I am well supported

**Steps I need to take to
achieve my goal**

To find out more

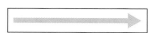

about clinical supervision

To start a

reflective diary

Figure 17.6 Personal action plan.

Risks

To laugh is to risk appearing the fool

To weep is to risk appearing sentimental

To reach out to another is to risk involvement

To expose feelings is to risk exposing your true self

To place your ideas, your dreams before a crowd is to risk their loss

To love is to risk not being loved in return

To live is to risk death

To hope is to risk despair

To try is to risk failure

But risks must be taken

Because the greatest hazard is to risk nothing

The person, who risks nothing, does nothings has nothing and is nothing

They may avoid suffering and sorrow but they cannot learn, feel, change,

Grow, love or live, chained by their certitudes

They are slaves; they have forfeited their freedom

Only a person who risks is truly free!

(Richard Rector 1991)

When you invest time in yourself – you will be looking after yourself. As a result, you will be more equipped to support your patients, colleagues and to 'bring comfort and hope'.

REFERENCES

Bond M, Holland S 1998 Skills of clinical supervision for nurses. Open University Press, Buckingham

Donne J In: Cohen (ed.) 1963 The Penguin dictionary of quotations. Penguin, Harmondsworth

McKenzie C 1994 Perfect stress control. Arrow Business Books, Essex

Murray Parkes C 1998 Coping with loss, the dying adult. BMJ Publications, London

Rector R 1991 Risks (unpublished work)

Sach P 1997 Take care of yourself. Penguin, Harmondsworth

Stotter D 1992 The culture of care. Nursing Times 88(12): 30–31

Sweetenham J 1997 Reflection in action model (unpublished work)

Twycross R 1995 Introducing palliative care. Radcliffe Medical Press, Oxford

Vachon M 1997 Recent research into staff stress in palliative care. European Journal of Palliative Care 4(3): 99–103

Williams S 1998 Improving the health of the NHS workforce. The Nuffield Trust, London

Wilson P 1996 The little book of calm. Penguin, Harmondsworth

Index